Food and Drink in Archaeology 1
University of Nottingham Postgraduate Conference 2007

Food and Drink in Archaeology I

University of Nottingham Postgraduate Conference 2007

Edited by
Sera Baker, Martyn Allen,
Sarah Middle and Kristopher Poole

Series Editors: Naomi Sykes and Claire Newton

Prospect Books
2008

First published in Great Britain in 2008 by Prospect Books, Allaleigh House, Blackawton, Totnes, Devon, TQ9 7DL.

© 2008 as a collection Prospect Books.
© 2008 in individual articles rests with the authors.

The authors assert their moral right to be identified as authors in accordance with the Copyright, Designs & Patents Act 1988. No part of this publication may be reproduced, stored in a retrieval system or transmitted in any form of by any means, electronic, mechanical, photocopying, recording or otherwise, without the prior permission of the copyright holders.

ISBN 978-1-903018-60-6

The illustration on the cover is of a set of medieval jugs, courtesy of the University of Nottingham Archaeology Museum.

For more information about Prospect Books: www.prospectbooks.co.uk.

Design and typesetting in Gill Sans and Adobe Garamond by Tom Jaine.
Printed and bound in Great Britain by The Cromwell Press, Trowbridge.

Contents

List of Figures	7
Preface *Sera Baker*	9
Intoxication and Initiation: Alcohol and the Cult of the Kabeiroi *Kirsten Bedigan*	11
Changing Tastes in Sixteenth-Century England: Evidence from the Household Accounts of the Willoughby Family *Mark Dawson*	20
An Invitation to War: Constructing Alliances and Allegiances through Mycenaean Palatial Feasts *Rachel Fox and Katherine Harrell*	28
'The Privilege of Civilization': Cultural Change at the Victorian Dining Table *Annie Gray*	38
Take it with a Pinch of Salt? Thinking About the Cultural Significance of Producing and Consuming Salt *Sarah-Jane Hathaway*	47
The Distribution of the Catering Trade in Ostia Antica *Anna Kieburg*	57
Medieval Diet: Evidence for a London Signature? *Kay Lakin*	65
New Temptations? Olive, Cherry and Mulberry in Roman and Medieval Europe *Alexandra Livarda*	73
Gathered Food Plants at Dutch Mesolithic and Neolithic Wetland Sites *Welmoed Out*	84
Dinner at the Edge of the World: Why the Greenland Norse Tried to Eat a European Diet in an Unforgiving Landscape *Elizabeth Pierce*	96
Living and Eating in Viking-Age Towns and their Hinterlands *Kristopher Poole*	104

Stable Isotope Analysis of Skeletal Remains from Jordan:
    Environment, Diet and Societies of Past Southern Levant   113
    Michela Sandias

Feasting and Subsistence in Early Medieval Ireland and Wales:
    An Examination of the Literary and Archaeological Evidence   122
    Anne Sassin

The Origins of the Archaic Greek *Symposium*:
    Internal Developments and Near Eastern Influences   131
    Karin Schuitema

Foodways as a Reflection of Cultural Identity in a Roman Frontier Province:
    Bridging the Gap from Theory to Material   141
    Aviva Shuman

The Pewsey Middens: Centres of Feasting or Symbols of Community?   149
    Andy Tullett and Chris Harrison

Shorter Contributions

Zooarchaeological Research in Apulia, Southern Italy: Some Considerations
    of Animal Exploitation from Late Antiquity to the Early Middle Ages   159
    Antonietta Buglione

A Social Zooarchaeology of Feasting: The Evidence
    from the Ritual Deposit at Nopigeia, Crete   163
    Kerry Harris and Yannis Hamilakis

Fourth-Century AD Glass Tablewares from the Small
    Bathhouse in Eleutherna-Sector I, Crete   165
    Kalliopi Nikita

Trout Processing in the Upper Palaeolithic?   167
    Hannah Russ, Randolph Donahue and Andrew Jones

'A People who Eat Wood and Drink Water, the Devil can not
    Persuade, nor can Man.' Food in Rural Areas During the
    Middle Ages (*ca.* AD 1050–1532) in County Dalarna, Sweden:
    An Example from Västannorstjärn   170
    Mikael Simonsson

List of Figures

1.1. Kabeiric sites in the Eastern Mediterranean, Black Sea and Egypt. 12
1.2. Chronological and proportional spread of drinking vessels. at the sanctuaries of the Kabeiroi and Great Gods. 14
1.3. Part of a scene depicting a possible initiation, Thebes. 15
3.1. Plan of the Palace of Nestor at Pylos. 29
3.2. Pylos tablet Un 718. 32
4.1. *Service à la Française* (Simpson 1807). 39
4.2. *Service à la Russe* (Marshall *ca.* 1888). 40
4.3. Osborne House provisioning ledger. 44
5.1. Diagram showing a method of coastal salt production. 48
5.2. The life-cycle of briquetage. 50
5.3. Uses of salt. 51
6.1. Map of ancient Ostia. 58
6.2. Ground plan of the Porticus of Hercules. 61
6.3. Rebuilt shelf element in tavern no. 28. 62
6.4. Hypothetical reconstruction of an additional counter element in tavern no. 28. 63
7.1. Isotopic map. 66
7.2. Human isotope data for six late-medieval sites, St Giles by Brompton Bridge, Warrington, Towton, St Andrews at Fishergate, Wharram Percy, Orkney and St Mary Spital. 70
8.1. Chronological distribution of waterlogged records of olive, cherry and mulberry. 76
8.2. Social access to olive, cherry and mulberry. 77
8.3. Geographical dispersal of waterlogged olive, cherry and mulberry. 78
8.4. Proportion of site types with waterlogged cherry. 79
8.5. Geographical dispersal of waterlogged cherry. 80
8.6. Geographical dispersal of waterlogged cherry and mulberry. 81
9.1. Palaeogeographic map of the Netherlands at 4200 cal BC. 85

11.1. Relative frequencies of main domesticates in north/east and south/west England.	105
11.2. Relative frequencies of cattle culled on Mid-Saxon and Viking-Age rural sites.	106
11.3. Relative frequencies of domestic birds in north/east and south/west England.	107
12.1. Map of Jordan.	116
12.2. Mean $\delta^{13}C$ and $\delta^{15}N$ ratios for Tell Ya'amun and Khirbet Yajuz.	118
14.1. Table illustrating different periods in the Near East and the Aegean.	130
14.2. Map of the Aegean and the Near East.	132
14.3. The three modes of élite feasts.	133
14.4. The concept of emulation related to the emergence of the reclining *symposium* in the Aegean.	137
14.5. The development of and influences on the Archaic Greek *symposium*.	138
15.1. Relative percentages of three main domesticates in military contexts in Nijmegen.	145
15.2. Relative percentages of three main domesticates in civilian contexts in Nijmegen.	146
15.3. Relative percentages of species found in cult complexes in Nijmegen.	147
16.1. Sheep mortality at Stanton St Bernard.	154
18.1. Cattle metapodia with distal ends broken off, Nopigeia, Crete.	162
18.2. Cattle metacarpal with hole in proximal end, Nopigeia, Crete.	162
20.1. The Fucino Basin today.	168
20.2. Fish remains in a one-year-old bear scat.	168
21.1. A woman making butter with the help of the Devil using high and low stave-built vessels.	171
21.2. Diagram showing the relative frequency of cattle, sheep/goat and pig remains at Västannorstjärn.	172

Preface

This volume is the first of what we trust will be a long series of proceedings deriving from the new annual Food and Drink in Archaeology conference. The inaugural conference was held on the 18 and 19 May 2007 at the University of Nottingham. It was conceived and organized by PhD students from this University's Department of Archaeology who were keen to provide a rare platform for post-graduate and early-career researchers to present and publish their work. Food and drink was a natural choice for the conference theme, being a topic both at the top of scholarly debate and of relevance to the study of all cultures, regardless of time and space. The wide appeal of the subject is reflected in this volume, which contains 21 papers (16 given as papers at the conference with five shorter articles composed from posters) transporting the reader across landscapes and cultures from the Levant to Greenland and from the Mesolithic to the Victorian periods.

The contents of this volume, offered by authors based in universities across Europe, are impressive; all adopt genuinely integrated approaches, weaving together evidence from multiple sources – material culture, zooarchaeology, archaeobotany, isotopic analysis, architecture, history and iconography – to answer questions about the production, distribution and consumption of food and drink. By so doing this volume provides an insight into the practices, ideology and identity of a range of past societies: the ancient Greeks, European Iron Age, Romans, Vikings and Tudors to name but a few.

On behalf of the organizing committee, I should like to thank the contributors of this volume and our publisher, Tom Jaine of Prospect Books, for his support and patience. Special thanks must go to the many anonymous reviewers who not only ensured the quality of the material contained within this volume but who also took the time to provide the contributors with invaluable advice; those of us who are publishing here for the first time are particularly grateful. Without the support of The University of Nottingham's School of Humanities, who granted us RCUK's Career Development and Skills Training for Research Students and Researchers Payments (Roberts Money), and The University of Nottingham's Alumni Fund, the initial conference and this volume would not have been possible.

Sera Baker,
University of Nottingham

Intoxication and Initiation: Alcohol and the Cult of the Kabeiroi

Kirsten Bedigan, University of Glasgow

Introduction
The function of feasting in ancient Greek religion is well testified (Burkert 2001, 107); however, the role of alcohol within the types of cults known as the mysteries is less clear. These cults, from the well-known Eleusinian mysteries of Demeter to the more obscure Kabeiric mysteries, performed ceremonies of initiation. The name 'mystery cult' derives from the premise that only the initiated were allowed access to its secrets. We know from literary evidence that an intoxicant known as *kykeon* played a role in the Eleusinian mysteries of Demeter (*Homeric Hymn to Demeter*, trans. Cashford and Richardson 2003, lines 197–212). Unfortunately little literary evidence exists for the Kabeiroi but it is clear that the cult was widespread (see Fig. 1) with over 90 Kabeiric sites across the eastern Mediterranean and even as far as India (Lehmann and Spitle 1964, 132). The iconography and archaeology facilitate an anthropological approach to the role of alcohol within the initiation rites of this cult.

Rites of Passage
A rite of passage is here defined as a ritual performance by which an individual moves from one socially-approved position into another. Bell (1997, 94) has suggested all rituals to be rites of passage and represent an exception to ordinary social practice. In the case of initiation, the rites of passage have three distinct phases. In stage one, the liminal phase, the initiate is removed from normal circumstances and purified in preparation for the rituals that are to follow (Burkert 2001, 75–77). For mystery religions, stage two is the separation phase, usually comprising the actual initiation. In the Eleusinian mysteries, which are relatively well documented despite the supposed secrecy of the cult, there were several events during initiation: a re-enactment or performance, presumably of the story of Demeter and Kore, the witnessing of sacred objects, and the recitation of prayers (Preka-Alexandri 2000, 20–21). Finally in the third stage, the aggregation phase, the initiate re-enters society as a member of the cult, with the good fortune that is bestowed upon them: salvation after death at the sanctuary of Eleusis (Burkert 2001, 289). Although the evidence for the activities of the Kabeiric cult is much rarer, the rituals, based upon the extant data, indicate that the cult operated in a similar manner.

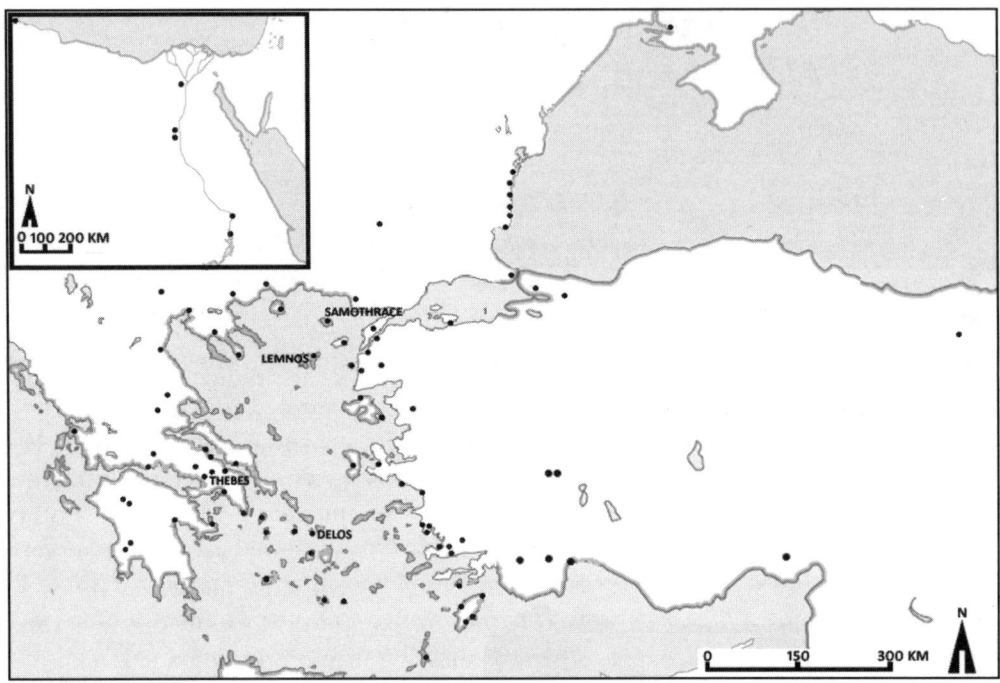

Figure 1.1. Kabeiric sites in the Eastern Mediterranean, Black Sea and Egypt, the case studies are named (image © K. Bedigan). Site identification based upon the following: Daumas 1998, Guettel-Cole 1984, Hemberg 1950, Herodotus Histories (trans. de Selincourt) 1996, and Schachter 1986.

Modern Anthropological Approaches: Teenage Drinking and Initiation

The mystery cult involved the initiation of individuals into a socially-bonded group that had no blood ties; no-one was excluded, with a few certain exceptions such as murderers (Schachter 1986, 96). The group dynamic of mystery cult initiates may be viewed as analogous to the modern-day fraternity houses, typically associated with American universities, where the practice of initiation, or 'hazing', exposes new potential recruits to 'a variety of challenges and situations…so that the brothers can evaluate the pledges' willingness to submit themselves to the organization' (Rhoads 1995, 312–13). Unlike a mystery cult where membership was fairly open, the fraternity retains the right to reject unsuitable candidates, creating a tiered system of status: those within the fraternity system, those who are outside of it and those who have sought entry but have been rejected.

The role of alcohol within the initiation rites of a fraternity is important. Initiates can be requested to participate in any activity the older brothers deem necessary and this includes the consumption of large quantities of alcohol (Nuwar 2001, 32). The transitional experience of an individual frequently corresponds to the consumption of intoxicants; alcohol is often an accompaniment to important stages within a person's life (Beccaria and Sande 2003, 101). In the case of the fraternity initiation, alcohol is a factor in the acceptance and integration of an individual into that society.

Alcohol and Ritual

Whilst alcohol consumption within a fraternity signals an individual's willingness to submit to the prescribed standards of a particular social group, intoxication in initiatory practices can have deeper, ritualistic interpretations. The three-stage rite of passage format, as described earlier, can be applied to the consumption of alcohol itself. The liminal phase can be associated with the first drink, separation with the period of intoxication, and aggregation when the alcohol is leaving or has left their system. The new identity associated with this stage can be reflected in the often rueful remembrance of activities performed whilst under the influence or on the current physical problems of detoxification – the hangover.

It is the intoxicative elements which make alcohol so important in particular events, 'its heightened social significance derives from…these psychoactive properties' (Dietler 1998, 310). Interpretations of the effects of this intoxication can be divided into two responses: first, that alcohol changes a person, allowing them to develop a new identity or tap into the subconscious (Giles 1999, 388). The second suggests that alcohol allows an individual to escape from themselves, to literally lose themselves in the intoxication (Giles 1999, 395). Whilst we know that alcohol can change people, for better or worse, how does this relate to the rituals of initiation? It would seem that intoxication is key. Lewis-Williams and Dowson (1993, 56) have proposed that there are stages of hallucination when a subject is intoxicated; these episodes may have enhanced the visual and aural stimulation that we know was part of the second and third phases of cultic initiation (Preka-Alexandri 2000, 20–21). Any object or phrase, however ordinary, shown or spoken to an intoxicated person accompanied by appropriate ritual, would seem to have elevated importance. Social conditioning would enable the initiate, even if the object or phrase was later forgotten, to apply this idea of knowledge to themselves. However, given that membership was a personal choice, it is important to remember that an individual would already have been willing to view the rituals as significant and that alcohol would merely heighten this emotion.

Material Culture of Alcohol and the Kabeiroi

The Kabeiric cult was more widespread than many supposed. Hemberg's (1950) volume *Die Kabiren* provided a catalogue to a large number of these sites. However, nearly 60 years of archaeological exploration have passed since the publication and the evidence suggests that Hemberg's work underestimated the size and importance of the cult. Unlike the Eleusinian mysteries, this particular cult has been largely overlooked by modern researchers and is consequently poorly understood. Given the aforementioned

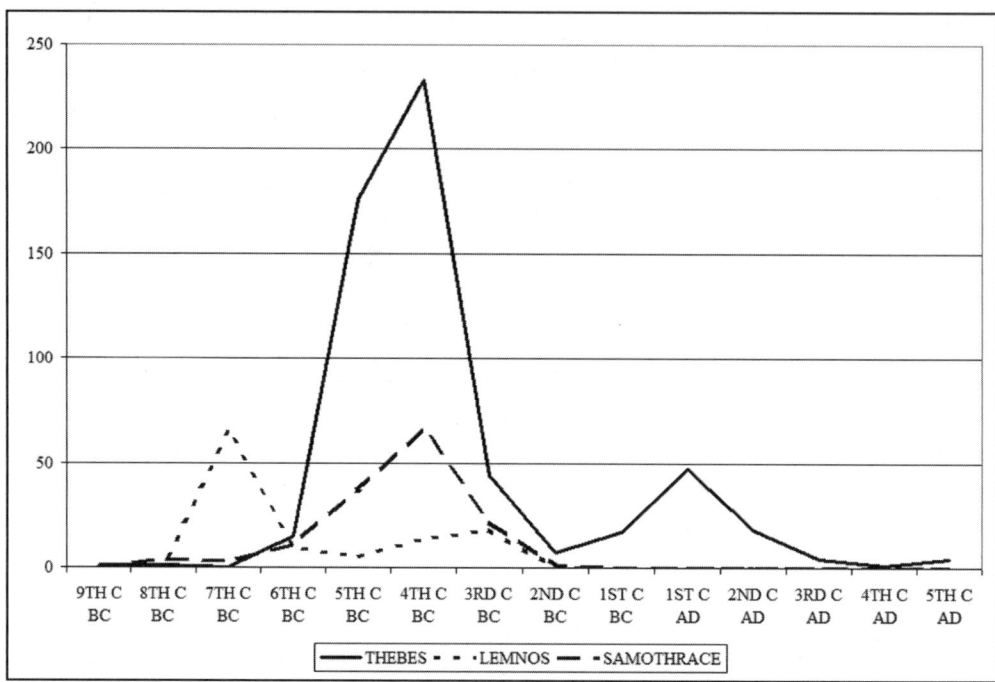

Figure 1.2. Chronological and proportional spread of drinking vessels at the sanctuaries of the Kabeiroi and Great Gods at Thebes, Lemnos and Samothrace. (Sources: Beschi 1997, 1998, 2003a, 2003b; Beschi et al. 2004; Bouzek et al. 1985; Braun and Haevernick 1981; Bruns 1964, 1967; Di Vita 1985, 1989, 1993; Gropengiesser 1970; Heimberg 1982; Kunisch 1971; Lehmann, K. 1960, 1962; Lehmann, K. and Spitle 1964; Lehmann, P.W. 1969; Lehmann, P.W. and Spitle 1982; Levi 1964; McCredie et al. 1992; Monaco and Monaco 2000; Myrina Archaeological Museum, Lemnos; National Archaeological Museum, Athens; Nicole 1911; Poggesi et al. 1997; Schauenberg 1954; Ure 1945, 1951; Ure Museum of Classical Art and Archaeology, Reading; Waiblinger 1974; Webster 1978; Wolters and Bruns 1940.)

lack of literary evidence, the archaeological data provide our only true insight into cult actions and activities.

From one of the few extant pieces of literature, a fragment of a lost play by Aeschylus, *The Kabeiroi*, we know that there was an obsession with alcohol and that this should be reflected in the material culture of a Kabeiric sanctuary. Unfortunately, despite the relative scale of the cult, archaeological data are not necessarily accessible. Out of the 94 identified sites, only four have been excavated and published: Thebes in central Greece, Lemnos and Samothrace in the North Aegean Islands, and Delos in the Cyclades (Fig. 1.1). The data used here are drawn from the ceramic finds from these sanctuaries, although there are lacunae in the information: for instance, the site report

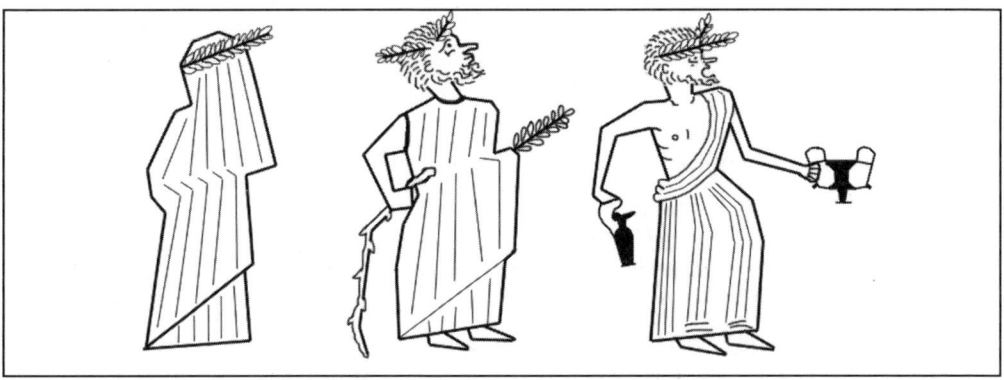

Figure 1.3. Part of a scene depicting a possible initiation from a late-fifth–early-fourth-century BC skyphos by the Mystes Painter found at the sanctuary of the Kabeiroi at Thebes. (Image © K. Bedigan; Wolters and Bruns 1940, 106 M2, Pl. 33.3; Braun and Haevernick 1981, 62 No. 292.)

for the Kabeirion on Delos presents no specific ceramic evidence (Chapouthier 1935, 80). The data from the remaining three sanctuaries are, however, significantly better. Thebes shows a marked increase in the number of vessels associated with drinking from the sixth century BC onwards before declining during the first century AD (Fig. 1.2). The peak in the fourth century can be linked specifically to the production of Kabeiric ware in Thebes. This local ceramic type was created only for the sanctuary of the Kabeiroi and consists of a grotesque-comic school of black figure decoration. The majority of the vessels produced in this style comprise drinking cups (especially the skyphos) and other alcohol-associated paraphernalia. Drinking paraphernalia also peaks in the fourth century BC at Samothrace, but Lemnos has a different pattern of development. Here, evidence for drinking practices appears at an early stage of the sanctuary's development, in the seventh century BC. Thereafter, evidence for drinking decreases, with a minor revival in the the fourth and third centuries BC, a characteristic shared with both Thebes and Samothrace.

Visual Evidence for Alcohol Use in Initiation into the Kabeiric Cult

Current interpretation of the iconographic evidence from the class of vessels known collectively as Kabeiric ware suggests that the images might reflect the initiation rituals, along with other activities, practised at the cult centre in Thebes (Schachter 1986, 100 n. 3). One particular vessel has been interpreted as a scene showing preparation for initiation. Running from left to right, the scene has a narrative quality (Fig. 1.3). At the far left a figure is shown robed entirely from head to toe; next a figure is carrying foliage, which may have a votive purpose. This is followed by perhaps the most interesting figure, depicted carrying a wine jug and drinking cup. The scene continues with a grotesquely drawn figure dancing, brandishing two flaming torches; at the right are two women carrying sashes, these appear to have a function within the cult as many figures are shown wearing them knotted about their heads.

If this scene does indeed show an initiation then the consumption of alcohol or another intoxicant must have been integral to the ceremony. We know from literary evidence relating to Eleusis that initiates re-enacted Demeter's fast following the abduction of her daughter Persephone, before consuming an intoxicant which represented her breaking the fast (*Homeric Hymn to Demeter* trans. Cashford and Richardson 2003, lines 197–212). The actual physical properties of the *kykeon* are not clear – it may be an intoxicant but likewise it could simply represent a basic foodstuff (Rosen 1987, 416). In Homer's *Iliad* (trans. Murray 1999, 11.624–641) the *kykeon* is just a simple food or drink. However, other references to the *kykeon* in the literary sources suggest that it may indeed have had an intoxicative effect. In Homer's *Odyssey* (trans. Murray and Dimock 1995, 10.234), Hermes warns Odysseus about the enchanting properties of Circe's potion. The creation of this *kykeon* is described (*ibid*, 10.234–5) and its contents sound fairly innocuous, with the exception of the drugs that Circe adds. It is again referred to when Circe offers Odysseus this drink (*ibid*, 10.316). Curiously this scene appears with regularity on the vases from the Kabeirion at Thebes. Since Eleusis had re-enactments it would seem quite possible that the Theban site did so as well. Seating arrangements at the sanctuary would facilitate large-scale entertainment although it is not possible to prove that this was the case (Schachter 2003, 130).

By combining the iconographic, archaeological and literary evidence available, it is clear that intoxication played a role in initiation. If we consider first the iconographic data from Thebes the majority of vessels depicted appear to be those associated with symposia or celebratory activities. However, a large number do belong to the category of preliminary events, activities and rituals performed before initiation into the cult. More importantly the types of vessels seen within the iconography are primarily concerned with the consumption of alcohol. The archaeological material from Thebes, Samothrace and Lemnos demonstrates a similar level of specialization, drinking paraphernalia comprising the largest category of ceramic evidence. Whilst part of the ceramic corpus is clearly derived from symposia or similar activities at the cult centres, it is also highly probable that some were used in more secretive rituals. The literature, although scant for the Kabeiric cult, does indicate a definite focus on the consumption of alcohol (Aeschylus, *Kabeiroi* trans. Weir Smith, 1957). The evidence from Eleusis suggests that intoxicants may have been incorporated into initiation re-enactments. If we consider this possibility more carefully for the Kabeiric cult, the tale of Circe and Odysseus (Homer, *Odyssey* trans. Murray and Dimock 1995, 10.234) would make a logical choice. This story promotes the idea of alcohol (or another intoxicant) as a tool for change, whether good or bad.

Conclusion

If indeed the *kykeon* 'alters one's psychological state' (Rosen 1987, 423), then what was the purpose of such intoxication within a religious context? As we saw in the anthropological studies of the American fraternity system, alcohol was an important factor in the testing and acceptance of new initiates. Likewise, in ancient Greece, wine was often used as a social tool to test personality: 'It is in fire that experts test gold and silver; it is wine that discloses the soul of man' (Theognis, quotation from Lissarrague 1987, 8). Modern studies have suggested that those who imbibed alcohol were influenced by those around them. If their social peer(s) told an individual that they were violent while drunk, this becomes a 'self-fulfilling prophecy' (Giles 1999, 389). The idea of alcoholic prophecy is useful; essentially it is a form of social-programming – establishing an idea in advance to gain the correct reaction when the intoxicated initiate is shown the secret rites. Alcohol affects personality (Lissarrague 1987, 10). Initiates can be stripped of individuality and programmed to behave in an appropriate manner. If we then assume alcohol plays a role in initiation we can argue that it is the very properties of this intoxicant which are so beneficial to the ceremony. In the initiation rites of the Kabeiric cult alcohol acted as a social liberator, stripping souls bare and allowing them to be reshaped to a form which suited the cult best even if it was only for the duration of the intoxication.

Bibliography

Beccaria, F. and Sande, A. 2003. 'Drinking games and rite of life projects: a social comparison of the meaning and functions of young people's use of alcohol during the rite of passage to adulthood in Italy and Norway', *Young: Nordic Journal of Youth Research* **11**, 99–119.

Bell, C. 1997. *Ritual: Perspectives and Dimensions* (Oxford).

Beschi, L. 1997. 'Un deposito de ceramiche tardoclassiche ed ellenistiche dal Cabirio de Lemno: considerazioni generali', in Archontidou-Argyri, A., Drougou, S., Zervoudaki, I., Marangou, L. and Touratsoglou, G. (eds) *D' Epistemonike sunantisi gia tin Ellinistiki Keramiki. Chronologika Provlimata Kleista Sunola-Ergastiria. Mytilini, Martios 1994* (Athens), 211–219.

Beschi, L. 1998. 'Arte e culture di Lemno arcaica', *La Parola del Passato. Rivista di Studi Antichi* **53**, 48–76.

Beschi, L. 2003a. 'Ceramiche archaice di Lemno: alcuni problemi', *Annuario della Scuola Archeologica de Atene e delle Missioni Italiene de Oriente* **81**, 303–349.

Beschi, L. 2003b. 'Il primitivo telesterio del Cabirio di Lemno (campagne di scavo 1990–1991)', *Annuario della Scuola Archeologica de Atene e delle Missioni Italiene Oriente* **81**, 963–994.

Beschi, L., Monaco, M.C., Zarkadas, A. and Gorini, G. 2004. 'Il telesterio ellenistico del Cabirio di Lemno', *Annuario della Scuola Archeologica de Atene e delle Missioni Italiene di Oriente* **82**, 225–341.

Bouzek, J., Ondřejová, I. and Hošek, R. 1985. *Samothrace 1923/1927/1978. The Results of the Czechoslovak Excavations in 1927 Conducted by A. Salač and J. Nepomucký and the Unpublished Results of the 1923 Franco-Czechoslovak Excavations Conducted by A. Salač and F. Chapouthier* (Prague).

Braun, K. and Haevernick, T. E. 1981. *Bemalte Keramik und Glas aus dem Kabirenheiligtum bei Theben* (Berlin).

Bruns, G. 1964. 'Kabirenheiligtum bei Theben. Vorläufiger bericht über die grabungskampagnen 1959 und 1962', *Archäologischer Anzeiger* **79**, 231–265.

Bruns, G. 1967. 'Kabirenheiligtum bei Theben. Vorläufiger bericht über die grabungskampagnen 1964–1966', *Archäologischer Anzeiger* **82**, 228–273.

Burkert, W. 2001. *Greek Religion* (Oxford).

Cashford, J. and Richardson, N. (trans.) 2003. *Homeric Hymn to Demeter* (London).

Chapouthier, F. 1935. *Le Sanctuarie des Dieux de Samothrace* (Paris).

Daumas, M. 1998. *Cabiriaca: Recherches sur l'Iconographie du Culte des Cabires* (Paris).

de Sélincourt, A. (trans.) 1996. *Herodotus, Histories* (London).

Di Vita, A. 1985. 'Atti della scuola 1985', *Annuario della Scuola Archeologica de Atene e delle Missioni Italiene Oriente* **63**, 337–377.

Di Vita, A. 1989. 'Atti della scuola 1988–1989', *Annuario della Scuola Archeologica de Atene e delle Missioni Italiene Oriente* **66–67**, 427–483.

Di Vita, A. 1993. 'Atti della scuola 1992–1993', *Annuario della Scuola Archeologica de Atene e delle Missioni Italiene Oriente* **70–71**, 395–486.

Dietler, M. 1998. 'Comment on A.H. Joffre, alcohol and social complexity in ancient western Asia', *Current Anthropology* **39**, 310–311.

Giles, D. 1999. 'Retrospective accounts of drunken behaviour: implications for theories of self, memory and discursive construction of identity', *Discourse Studies* **1**, 387–403.

Gropengiesser, H. 1970. *Corpus Vasorum Antiquorum. Heidelberg, Universität 4, Deutschland 31* (Munich).

Guettel-Cole, S. 1984. *Theoi Megaloi: The Cult of the Great Gods at Samothrace* (Leiden).

Heimberg, U. 1982. *Die Keramik des Kabirions* (Berlin).

Hemberg, B. 1950. *Die Kabiren* (Uppsala).

Kunisch, N. 1971. *Corpus Vasorum Antiquorum. Berlin, Antiquarium 4, Deutschland 33* (Munich).

Lehmann, K. 1960. *Samothrace: Excavations Conducted by the Institute of Fine Arts of New York University. Volume II, Part II. The Inscriptions on Ceramics* (London).

Lehmann, K. 1962. *Samothrace: Excavations Conducted by the Institute of Fine Arts of New York University. Volume IV, Part I. The Hall of Votive Gifts* (London).
Lehmann, K. and Spitle, D. 1964. *Samothrace: Excavations conducted by the Institute of Fine Arts of New York University. Volume IV, Part II. The Altar Court* (London).
Lehmann, P. W. 1969. *Samothrace: Excavations conducted by the Institute of Fine Arts of New York University. Volume III, Part II. The Hieron* (London).
Lehmann, P. W. and Spitle, D. 1982. *Samothrace: Excavations conducted by the Institute of Fine Arts of New York University. Volume V, Part I. The Temenos* (Princeton).
Levi, P. 1964. 'Il Cabirio di Lemno', *Charistirion eis anastasion k. oplandon. Dimosieuma tis Athinais Archaiologikis etaireias* **G**, 110–132.
Lewis-Williams, J. D. and Dowson, T. A. 1993. 'On vision and power in the Neolithic: evidence from the decorated monuments', *Current Anthropology* **34**, 55–65.
Lissarrague, F. 1987. *The Aesthetics of the Greek Banquet: Images of Wine and Ritual, Un Flot d'Images* (Princeton).
McCredie, J. R., Roux, G., Shaw, S. M. and Kurtich, J. 1992. *Samothrace: Excavations Conducted by the Institute of Fine Arts of New York University. Volume VII, Part I. The Rotunda of Arsinoe* (Princeton).
Monaco, M. C. and Monaco, M. Ch. 2000. 'Un deposito di ceramiche tardoclassiche ed ellenistiche dal Cabirio di Lemno: analisi delle forme II: ceramica acroma e da cucina', in Kypraiou, E. (ed.) *E' Epistemonike sunantisi gia tin Ellinistiki Keramiki. Praktika – Chania, Aprilios 1997. Chronologika provlimata. Kleista Sunola-Ergastiria. Keimena* (Athens), 153–160.
Murray A. T. (trans.) 1999. *Homer, The Iliad* (Cambridge, Massachusetts).
Murray, A. T. and Dimock, G. E. (trans.) 1995. *Homer, The Odyssey* (Cambridge, Massachusetts).
Nicole, G. 1911. *Catalogue des Vases Peints du Musée National d'Athènes* (Paris).
Nuwar, H. 2001. *Wrongs of Passage: Fraternities, Sororities, Hazing and Binge Drinking* (Bloomington).
Poggesi, G., Savona, S., Monaco, M. Ch. and Monaco, M. C. 1997. 'Un deposito di ceramiche tardoclassiche ed ellenistiche dal Cabiro di Lemno: analisi delle forme', in Archontidou-Argyri, A., Drougou, S., Zervoudaki, I., Marangou, L. and Touratsoglou, G. (eds) *D' Epistemonike sunantisi gia tin Ellinistiki Keramiki. Chronologika Provlimata Kleista Sunola-Ergastiria. Mytilini, Martios 1994* (Athens), 220–231.
Preka-Alexandri, K. 2000. *Eleusis* 3rd Edn. (Athens).
Rhoads, R. M. 1995. 'Whales' tales, dog piles, and beer goggles: an ethnographic case study of fraternity life', *Anthropology and Education Quarterly* **26**, 306–323.
Rosen, R. M. 1987. 'Hipponax Fr.48 Dg. and the Eleusinian kykeon', *American Journal of Philology* **3**, 416–426.
Schachter, A. 1986. *Cults of Boeotia 2: Herakles to Poseidon* (London)
Schachter, A. 2003. 'Evolution of a mystery cult: the Theban Kabeiroi', in Cosmopoulos, M. B. (ed.) *Greek Mysteries: The Archaeology and Ritual of Ancient Greek Secret Cults* (London).
Schauenberg, K. 1954. *Corpus Vasorum Antiquorum: Heidelberg, Universität 1, Deutschland 10* (Munich).
Ure, A.D. 1945. 'Some provincial black-figure workshops', *Annual of the British School at Athens* **41**, 22–28.
Ure, A. D. 1951. 'Koes', *Journal of Hellenic Studies* **71**, 194–197.
Waiblinger, A. 1974. *Corpus Vasorum Antiquorum: Paris, Musée du Louvre 17, France 26* (Paris).
Webster, T. B. L. 1978. *Monuments illustrating Old and Middle Comedy* 3rd Edn., BICS Supplement 39 (London).
Weir Smith, H. (trans.) 1957. *Aeschylus, Kabeiroi* (Cambridge).
Wolters, P. and G. Bruns 1940. *Das Kabirenheiligtum bei Theben* (Berlin).

Changing Tastes in Sixteenth-Century England: Evidence from the Household Accounts of the Willoughby Family

Mark Dawson,
University of Nottingham

Introduction

The accounts kept by large lay and ecclesiastic households are frequently used by historians of the medieval period to reconstruct patterns of food provisioning and consumption (Woolgar 1999; Threlfall-Holmes 2005). These sources provide details of seasonal changes in these patterns as well as of changes over decades, suggesting subtle, but nonetheless important shifts in taste and in the availability of certain foods. This information is often difficult to gather from other historical sources and the archaeological record, which are more adept at producing the long view, charting changes over centuries.

With reference to the early-modern period, household accounts have been mined for information on a number of social and cultural topics, but to date there has been no systematic examination of household accounts for the data they contain on changing patterns of food provision and consumption. Thirsk (2007), in her book, *Food in Early Modern England*, makes use of examples from household accounts and other sources to chart changes in diet from 1500–1760. The ambitious scope of this work, however, covering regional and social patterns of diet over more than two centuries, leaves, as Thirsk (2007, *xviii*) says, 'pathways that others will follow in the future'. This paper presents a limited selection of findings from my own research into the household accounts of the Willoughby family, of Wollaton, Nottinghamshire and Middleton, Warwickshire, offering comparisons to Thirsk's more general conclusions, as well as those of other historians and archaeologists working on food and diet in the late-medieval and early-modern periods.

The accounts of the Willoughby family (hereafter cited as Middleton) offer a view of domestic life in a gentry household in the sixteenth century, covering most decades from the 1520s through to the early 1600s, making the archive a peculiarly rich and valuable source. They show patterns of food provision and consumption not just for the family but for their servants as well, suggesting changes in diet that were potentially experienced by other households and individuals across the Midlands. The accounts are not without their limitations, being mainly concerned with purchases whereas details on the consumption of dairy foods, vegetables and fruit are largely absent, a defect shared by many similar accounts (Dyer 1997, 115–22). The exact numbers and composition of the household also present an issue. In general, throughout the period studied, the household seems to have consisted of around 40 to 50 people, the overwhelming majority of whom were servants of various degrees (Dawson 2007, 33–4). Some servants, however, had their own households and may have returned there before supper, whilst others would often be away on business. In their place were visiting tradesmen and the servants of neighbouring families, either on business or accompanying their masters and mistresses, guests of the Willoughbys. It is hard to discount the possibility, therefore, that some of the changes described in this article were due to particular changes in household composition or habits; only further research will bear out whether they reflect wider regional or national patterns.

Ale and Beer

Arguably the most important dietary change in the sixteenth century was the shift from ale to beer as the main drink. Beer, brewed with hops, had been known in England since at least the fifteenth century, but it was only during the sixteenth century that it began to replace ale as the national drink, spreading gradually from London and the south-east out to the Midlands and eventually the north (Unger 2004, 101–2).

Year of Account	Location	Drink Brewed
29 Sep. 1547 – 29 Sep. 1548	Middleton	47795 litres beer 7154 litres ale
31 Mar. – 14 Dec. 1588	Wollaton	41496 litres beer 411 litres ale
16 Apr. 1598 – 20 Jan. 1599	Middleton	45947 litres beer
12 Aug. 1599 – 3 May 1600	Wollaton	36352 litres beer 2470 litres strong beer

Table 2.1. Brewing at Middleton and Wollaton. (Source: Middleton, MiA27; MiA69; MiA74; MiA76.)

In the Willoughby household, ale was purchased regularly in the 1520s, by Henry Willoughby and his companions when on hunting trips, as well as for the household and for workers. In 1522, however, purchases of hops recorded in the Middleton accounts indicate that the household may have been brewing beer at this date (Middleton MiA16, ff.8–10). In the main, the household appears to have brewed its own drink and by 1547–8, the majority of that drink was beer, brewed invariably from malted barley. As table 2.1 shows, the accounts for Middleton for this year reveal that around 90 per cent of the drink brewed was beer. Later accounts suggest that the move to beer continued, perhaps as the last of the old ale-drinking retainers died off. In 1588 at Wollaton only one per cent of the drink brewed was ale and in 1598–9 at Middleton and 1599–1600 at Wollaton no ale was brewed or purchased at all.

The Willoughby household may have been in advance of other households in the local area in their conversion to beer drinking. During the 1560s, when the management of the estates was in the hands of executors, there are interesting glimpses of what may have been residual preferences for ale. At Wollaton, in July 1562, for example, sheep-shearers, who may have hailed from the north, were given ale. In the same year the auditors also drank ale, the remainder being sold to local colliers. At another audit later the same year, however, the purchase of 5lb (2.3kg) of hops suggests beer was drunk and at Middleton in 1567 tenants performing labour services were rewarded with beer (Middleton MiA42, ff.2v, 6v, 11; MiA55, f.7). Thomas Cogan (1589, 217) believed ale to be still common in rural areas of northern England, although it had been generally replaced by beer in urban areas and in wealthy households. It seems likely that a generation or so earlier, a similar situation had existed in the Midlands.

Meat

The main meat consumed within the household appears to have been beef. In 1547–8 at Middleton it represented around 40 per cent by weight of all the meat from domestic animals and a similar proportion in 1598–9 (Dawson 2007, 87). The predominance of beef accords with the comment of Thomas Cogan (1589, 113) who said that beef 'of all flesh is most usuall among English men'. For the monks of Durham Cathedral Priory in the late-fifteenth and early-sixteenth centuries, beef represented around 65 per cent of all the meat they consumed (Threlfall-Holmes 2005, 50). Mutton was generally the second most common meat; however, in rural areas, outside of large households, the situation could have been reversed due to the difficulties of disposing of an entire beef carcass at once. The predominance of beef may have been a feature of the diet in wealthy households rather than that of the nation as a whole (Albarella 1999, 869–72; Thirsk 2007, 237).

Within the Willoughby household, although beef seems to have remained dominant during the sixteenth century, there were changes in the proportions of other meats consumed, some of which are shown in table 2.2. Veal is rarely mentioned in the accounts from the 1520s and it was not purchased at all during Henry Willoughby's stay in London

	29 Sep. 1547 – 29 Sep. 1548	31 Mar. – 14 Dec. 1588	16 Apr. 1598 – 20 Jan. 1599	12 Aug. 1599 – 3 May 1600
Veal calves	21.5	30.5	38.2	24.3
Mature pigs	15	4.5	8.6	28.5
Young pigs	301	57	45	40
Chickens	746	271	133	180
Capons	200	103	71	174

Table 2.2. *Meat provision of selected whole animals. (Source: Middleton, MiA27; MiA69; MiA74; MiA76.)*

during April and May 1522, when his servants bought beef, mutton, lamb, chickens, rabbits and pigeons (Middleton, MiA10). However, in 1547–8, 21.5 veal carcasses were consumed at Middleton, and from April 1598 to January 1599 the figure was just over 38 carcasses. Considering that veal was mainly consumed between spring and early autumn, the figure of 24.3 carcasses for the household at Wollaton from August 1599 to April 1600 is also quite sizeable. The increase in veal consumption in the Willoughby household is reflected in archaeological studies of urban sites from the post-medieval period (Dobney *et al.* 1996, 31). The taste for veal could have been a consequence, or perhaps a stimulus, of the general increase in dairying noted within England as a whole in the late sixteenth and seventeenth centuries (Thirsk 2007, 46, 122).

At the same time as this increase in veal consumption there was an apparent decline in the importance of pig meat within the Willoughby household. This is a general trend observed in household accounts and archaeological evidence from the medieval period (Woolgar 1999, 134; Albarella 2006, 74, 77). Alongside the general decline, there was a change in the type of pig meat being consumed, with an increasing proportion of meat being supplied from fattened animals; porketts, brawns and bacons. Assuming the carcass weight of a young pig to be around a quarter that of a mature fattened animal (Harvey 1993, Appendix II), the figures for 1547–8 suggest that over 80 per cent of pig meat consumed in the household came from young pigs. That figure was around 50 per cent in 1598–9 and only around a quarter in 1599–1600. The account for 1599–1600 shows that porketts, bacon and brawn were consumed from October through to the weeks immediately after Lent, a pattern also visible for the porketts eaten at Middleton 1547–8. Had the accounts for 1588 and 1598–9 been carried through until the following Lent, the total number of mature pigs consumed would undoubtedly have been significantly higher.

Shifts in the type of pig meat being consumed also marked a change in the way that pigs were supplied to the household. Most of the 301 young pigs eaten in 1547–8 were bought and the caterer's account for Wollaton for March 1542 to March 1543 records a total of 365 young pigs purchased (Middleton, MiA25). The porketts consumed in 1547–8, on the other hand, were all supplied from the dairy at Middleton, as apparently were those eaten in 1598–9. The vast majority of the porketts eaten at Wollaton in 1599–1600 were listed as 'store' items, implying that they had come from the home farms.

A parallel change can also be detected in the provision and consumption of poultry within the household. Accounts from the 1520s show that large numbers of chickens were purchased – over 1000 in 1522 and 1524 (Middleton, MiA8, MiA9, MiA13, MiA14). Later accounts, however, reveal much smaller numbers of chickens being purchased and a greater proportion of fattened capons, many apparently supplied from the Willoughbys' own farms or by their tenants as gifts. In 1588, 46 out of 103 capons were listed under 'store', indicating that they potentially came from the home farm, whilst in 1599–1600, most of the poultry supplied to the household seems to have come in the form of gifts at Christmas and New Year (Middleton, MiA69, MiA76). Changes in the provision of both pigs and poultry suggest moves towards more specialist products, perhaps a reflection of shifting preferences within the social élite or a more widespread change in taste.

Fish

The provision and consumption of fish within the Willoughby household reveal a number of interesting and illustrative points. Fasting regulations remained in force throughout the sixteenth century, despite the religious changes brought by the Reformation. The protestant Edwardian and Elizabethan regimes gave the preservation of livestock numbers and support for the fishing industry as the ostensible reasons for maintaining, largely intact, the series of fasts inherited from the medieval Catholic Church (*Great Britain* 1786, 426, 539). Of course, fasting merely meant abstaining from meat and not necessarily eating fish; dairy foods were another alternative. However, in practice fasting during the sixteenth century generally meant the replacement of meat in the diet by fish.

Date of Purchase	Quantity Purchased
September 1524	120 'grett' ling and 180 lobbe (pollack)
September 1573	60 small ling, 60 large ling and 210 haberden
September 1588	150 ling and 150 salt cod
September 1599	138 ling and 124 haberden

Table 2.3. *Purchases of salted white fish at Stourbridge Fair. (Source: Middleton, MiA15; MiA57; MiA69; MiA76.)*

The vast majority of fish provided for the Willoughby household was preserved, fresh fish being an expensive luxury (Dawson 2007, 136–7; Woolgar 1999, 120–1). There were basically two main types of preserved fish: various forms of salted white fish (ling, cod, haberden and pollack), which were eaten as a staple on fast days throughout the year, and preserved herring (smoked red herring or pickled white herring), which were eaten during Lent. The Willoughbys, like many other large households, purchased their salted white fish in bulk at Stourbridge Fair, held near Cambridge in September. A sample of these bulk purchases, shown in table 2.3, reveals no appreciable decline in the overall amount of fish purchased, and throughout the sixteenth century saltfish would appear to have retained its place in the diet of the household as a whole. Fines could be levied on householders for every person within their own household who broke the fasting regulations and this seems to have been largely effective (*Great Britain* 1786, 665). However, although the fasts were strictly maintained at Middleton in 1547–8, during Francis Willoughby's visit to Wollaton in March 1587 two capons and a veal pie were consumed. In March 1600, a dinner held at Wollaton for the judges at Nottingham assizes included beef, brawn, mutton, veal, capons and woodcock, together with more appropriate Lenten fare: eels, carp, bream, perch and ling. The accounts for Middleton 1598–9 and Wollaton 1599–1600 also show the regular consumption of small quantities of mutton and poultry on Fridays and Saturdays (Middleton, MiA27, MiA69, MiA74, MiA76). This suggests that the master and mistress of the household, Percival and Bridget Willoughby, were prepared to break the fast, seemingly with the connivance of the local legal establishment, even if they were not prepared to risk having to pay for their servants to do the same thing.

Whilst the quantity of salted white fish purchased for the household seems to have remained roughly the same, the quantity of preserved herring declined markedly through the sixteenth century. Preserved herring were mainly consumed during Lent, when they were eaten in large quantities, supplemented by the usual salted white fish. Over 5000 herring were purchased for the household of Henry Willoughby in preparation for Lent 1524. In Lent 1548 the household at Middleton consumed around 3500 herring. By Lent 1587 just over 2000 herring were eaten by Francis Willoughby's household, and at Wollaton during Lent 1600, only around 1000 (Middleton, MiA15, MiA27, MiA69, MiA76). The decline in herring consumption can also be traced in medieval household accounts (Woolgar, 2000, 44); however, the impact of the Reformation seems to have exacerbated the situation, providing the occasion to ditch an increasingly unpopular food. Nevertheless, its place in the diet of the household had to be filled, and whilst the head of the household was seemingly prepared to break the fast, punitive measures appear to have been enough to prevent a more widespread flouting of the regulations. It seems probable that increased consumption of dairy foods would have filled this gap.

Dried Fruit and Spices

Grocery items – dried fruit and spices – were, like preserved fish, usually bought in bulk by the Willoughbys in the sixteenth century, and records of these purchases reveal subtle changes during the period. A sample of these figures is shown in tables 2.4 and 2.5, the figures for 1599–1600 representing only nine months but including the bulk purchase made at Lenton Fair. The quantity of dried fruit purchased seems to have increased towards the end of the century, reflecting perhaps the growing taste for fresh fruit. By contrast the quantity of spices purchased declined over the period, and there was also a reduction in their variety, with galingale, spikenard and long pepper, all bought at Lenton Fair in 1523 and 1524, no longer mentioned in the later accounts (Middleton, MiA11, f.20; MiA15, f.7). These figures are interesting in relation to the perceived general decrease in the use of spices in the high cuisine of continental Europe during the early-modern period (Flandrin 1999, 407–8), and the increasing prominence of fruit and vegetables, remarked upon by William Harrison (1994, 264) in the diet of his Elizabethan contemporaries. This suggests a move away from the highly spiced cuisine of the late-medieval period to what might be described as a more 'fruity' Elizabethan one.

	1523	1524	1573	1574	1599–1600
Almonds	17.3kg	4.9kg	2.7kg	2.7kg	1.1kg
Prunes	5.7kg	8.6kg	12.7kg	12.7kg	18.2kg
Raisins	2.7kg	3.2kg	6.4kg	14.1kg	10.5kg
Currants	5.5kg	18.2kg	12.7kg	25.5kg	23.2kg
Dates	-	-	3.2kg	-	-
Figs	-	-	-	-	0.9kg
Totals	31.2kg	34.9kg	37.7kg	55kg	43.9kg

Table 2.4. *Dried fruit purchased. (Source: Middleton, MiA11; MiA13; MiA57; MiA76.)*

	1523	1524	1573	1574	1599–1600
Pepper	13.6kg	17kg	7.3kg	13.6kg	3.6kg
Cinnamon	1.4kg	18kg	5.5kg	0.7kg	0.3kg
Ginger	3.8kg	4.1kg	2.7kg	2.7kg	0.6kg
Cloves	1.4kg	2.3kg	1.4kg	1.4kg	0.2kg
Mace	1kg	0.9kg	0.9kg	0.7kg	0.2kg
Nutmeg	0.1kg	0.3kg	1.8kg	1.8kg	0.5kg
Others	1.9kg	3.3kg	-	-	-
Totals	23.2kg	29.7kg	19.6kg	20.9kg	5.4kg

Table 2.5. *Spices purchased. (Source: Middleton, MiA11; MiA13; MiA57; MiA76.)*

Additionally, the mention of olives and capers in the accounts from the 1570s onwards points perhaps to an increasing Mediterranean influence (Middleton, MiA57, ff.10, 77; MiA71, f.78). In this light it is interesting to note that many of the architectural details included in new Wollaton Hall, begun in 1580, were of Italianate design. Neither Francis Willoughby's house nor his diet could be said to truly reflect Italian style – both were an amalgam – but they reveal, in contrast to those of his predecessors, the changes in taste that had occurred in sixteenth-century England.

Conclusion

This brief summary of dietary change in the Willoughby household during the sixteenth century should cause us to consider the influence of various factors upon the type of food and drink consumed. Agrarian and general economic changes undoubtedly had a great impact. Beer was more economical in its use of grain than ale and this was undoubtedly a factor in its increasing popularity in an era of growing population and rising grain prices. The religious and political effects of the English Reformation also left their mark, if not perhaps in the straightforward manner traditionally imagined. Legal strictures ensured that fasting was not a dead letter in Elizabethan England but the removal of the threat of damnation must surely have altered attitudes and seems to have accelerated the decline in the consumption of herring. Increased dairy production, witnessed by increased veal consumption, could have provided suitable alternatives for fast-days. But in this and in other changes it is important not to forget the role of personal taste. The decline in the consumption of both ale and preserved herring was gradual, probably resulting in differences in dietary habits between generations as well as between social groups. The gentry household of the Willoughbys was by no means representative of other households in the Midlands; nevertheless, the changes witnessed in that household could well have been repeated in the households of servants, who worked and ate in the hall during the day, and were introduced to dietary changes, new foods and new tastes. Perhaps the one thing we can say for sure is that diet in the sixteenth century, as today, was not static.

References

MANUSCRIPT SOURCES

University of Nottingham, Department of Manuscripts and Special Collections, Middleton MSS.

PRINTED SOURCES

Albarella, U. 1999. 'The mystery of husbandry; medieval animals and the problem of integrating historical and archaeological evidence', *Antiquity* **73**, 867–75.

Albarella, U. 2006. 'Pig husbandry and pork consumption in medieval England', in Woolgar, C.M., Serjeantson, D. and Waldron, T. (eds) *Food in Medieval England: Diet and Nutrition* (Oxford), 72–87.

Cogan, T. 1589. *The Haven of Health* (London).

Dawson, M. 2007. *Plenti and Grase: Food and Drink in a Sixteenth-Century Gentry Household*. Unpublished PhD thesis, University of Nottingham (Prospect Books, forthcoming).

Dobney, K., Jacques, D. and Irving, B. 1996. *Of Butchers and Breeds: Report on Vertebrate Remains from Various Sites in the City of Lincoln* (London).

Dyer, C. 1997. 'Do household accounts provide an accurate picture of late medieval diet and food culture?', in Rassart-Eeckhout, E., Sosson, J. P., Thiry, C. and van Hemelryck T. (eds) *La Vie Materielle au Moyen Age: L'Apport des Sources Litteraires, Normatives et de la Pratique* (Louvain-le-Neuve), 115–22.

Flandrin, J. L. 1999. 'Dietary choices and culinary technique', in Flandrin, J. L. and Montanari, M. (eds) *Food: A Culinary History from Antiquity to the Present* (New York), 403–17.

Great Britain 1786. *The Statutes at Large, From the First Year of the Reign of Edward the Fourth to the End of the Reign of Queen Elizabeth, Volume the Second* (London).

Harrison, W. 1994. *The Description of England* (New York).

Thirsk, J. 2007. *Food in Early Modern England: Phases, Fads, Fashions 1500–1760* (London).

Harvey, B. 1993. *Living and Dying in England 1100–1540: The Monastic Experience* (Oxford).

Threlfall-Holmes, M. 2005. *Monks and Markets: Durham Cathedral Priory 1460–1520* (Oxford).

Unger, R.W. 2004. *Beer in the Middle Ages and the Renaissance* (Philadelphia).

Woolgar, C.M. 1999. *The Great Household in Late Medieval England* (London).

Woolgar, C.M. 2000. '"Take this penance now, and afterwards the fare will improve"; seafood and late medieval diet', in Starkey, D. J., Reid, C. and Ashcroft, N. (eds) *England's Sea Fisheries: The Commercial Sea Fisheries of England and Wales since 1300* (London), 36–44.

An Invitation to War: Constructing Alliances and Allegiances through Mycenaean Palatial Feasts

Rachel Fox and Katherine Harrell,
University of Sheffield

Feasting as a Strategy

In recent years, Aegean prehistorians have recognized that the Mycenaean palaces served as arenas for large-scale feasting events and subsequently there has been a significant increase in the number of studies considering what might have been the purposes of these feasts: from celebrations of religious festivals to demonstrations of the *wanax*'s (the ruler's) authority. It is impossible to find one explanation that satisfactorily covers the variety of commensal occasions testified both in the archaeological and the textual evidence. However, with this caveat in mind, we will here propose that one of several reasons for hosting large-scale feasts in a palatial context was the potential mobilization of Mycenaean troops. It seems probable that this could have been an effective way of binding future soldiers to the palace's authority, and it undoubtedly was a straightforward method of ensuring the presence of large numbers of people in one defined place, with the consequent opportunity to manipulate the guests' obligations.

While feasting can generate feelings of community solidarity, it can also provide a channel for diffusing open aggression or concealing it under a façade of friendly commensality. The well-known north-western American potlatches reveal clearly how feasting and aggression can manifest an uneasy relationship, taken to an extreme by the Kwakiutl, whose rivalry-feasts involved violent destruction of property and escalated until one party was bankrupted (see Perodie 2001, 209). Even when less explicitly belligerent, feasting can exhibit a competitive nature that links it to aggression and the sphere of warfare, such as in south New Guinea where ceremonial food exchanges and feasting are a direct, mutually agreed substitute for warfare (Lemonnier 1996, 226).

This potential underlying association between feasting and warfare is made more explicit in cases of feasts in the ethnographic record whose purpose was to obtain allies. This need not be in the context of outright warfare, and may be to seek alliances in the event of future threat or to gain political allies who may prove advantageous to the sponsor. For example, the Tee cycle of feasts amongst the Enga in Papua New Guinea was employed, *inter alia*, as a method of attracting allies in or for warfare (Wiessner 2001, 122).

While feasts are often social and/or political in nature, a frequently attested economic goal in hosting them is that of mobilizing labour (Dietler and Herbich 2001, 242), where the host's generosity in food provision operates as a form of exchange for the guests' labour. It is sometimes difficult to acknowledge the frequency and power of

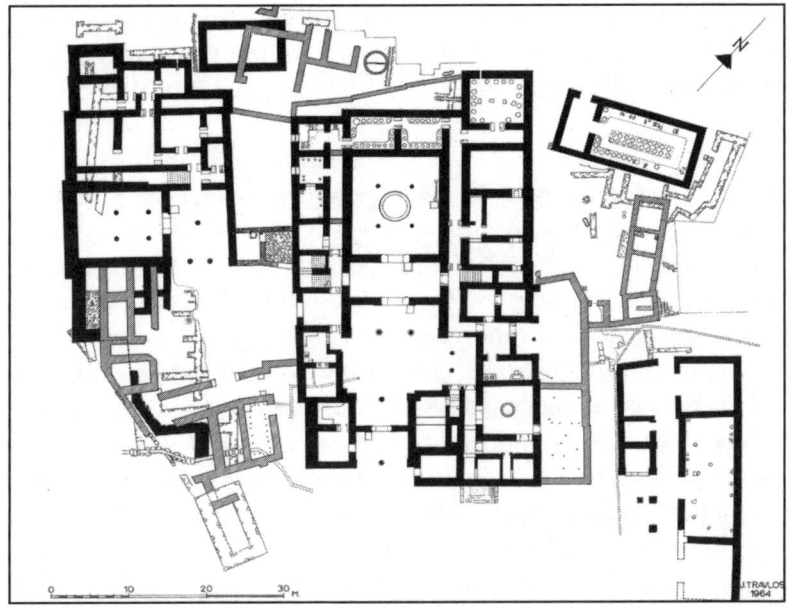

Figure 3.1. Plan of the Palace of Nestor at Pylos (after Blegen and Rawson 1966).

these collective work-events in harnessing a large labour force for the sponsor without any recompense beyond a good meal, and yet feasting was one of the principal means by which labour was mobilized for large-scale projects before the inception of a modern, Western monetary economy (Dietler and Herbich 2001, 240). Many of these feasts are voluntary in nature; the workers are attracted by the prospect of an extensive meal and a host with a reputation for generosity can harness the labour he requires without difficulty. However, the possibility remains that these occasions can become events of concealed exploitation. If it arises that only one sector of society or one person in the form of a leader can afford to sponsor large-scale feasts, then they can turn this system to their advantage. The opportunity therefore exists for a powerful, aggressive host to mobilize another form of labour through feasting, that of military service.

Obligations are created in feasting contexts through the conspicuous generosity of the host, which generates debts amongst the guests. These can be repaid in a variety of ways. At the most basic level, the guests could be obligated to invite their host back for a reciprocal meal. If, however, the power balance between guests and host is asymmetrical, then it may be that the guests are unable to reciprocate in kind, not having the available resources to equal or exceed the original feast. Thus they will be obligated to provide the host with labour or service in a form of gift exchange. In the case of diacritical feasts (see Dietler 2001, 85–8), inequality of status between host and guests is reinforced by a variety of methods; for example by serving guests with vessels that are noticeably poorer than those used by the host and his élite circle, or with lesser grades of cuisine supplied to those of inferior status. Therefore, not only would the guests be unable to pay the host back in kind, but they would realize how inherently inferior they were to him and potentially be more accepting of the demands placed on them in the name of reciprocity.

Feasting at Pylos

So far we have discussed the issue in generic and theoretical terms and we will now examine Mycenaean feasting specifically. There is clear evidence for the diacritical nature of feasts held in the Mycenaean palaces and marked divisions between social levels exhibited amongst the guests. This is an issue that has been discussed in detail by Bendall (2004) in relation to the palace at Pylos (Fig. 3.1), so we will summarize her arguments briefly. The uppermost level of élites dined in hall 6, the megaron, an enclosed and restricted area in the palace's heart, employing vessels of precious metal. A lower level of élites also dined in a restricted area, hall 65, which was towards the periphery of the palace, and used ceramic fineware vessels. The same ceramic fineware was used by the more general guests, who sat outside in courts 63/88. Finally, Bendall (2004, 123–4) has suggested a further level in those who sat outside the palace's entrance in court 58 and used ceramic semi-coarseware. It is also extremely likely that there was cuisine differentiation in the species or cuts of meat served to the general guests and to the host's circle and in the way they were prepared, although this requires more subtle interpretation of the archaeological record (Wright 2004, 40–1; Hruby 2006, 162–4). Thus it is clear that diacritica of various kinds were operative during palatial feasts; hence each guest must have been aware of their place in the social system, and the fact that perhaps the only chance they had of satisfactorily repaying their hosts was with some service that they could offer.

However, this fact does not distinguish between labour and military service and so it is worth examining the palatial feasts more closely to understand how they functioned. At Pylos, where the majority of our feasting evidence is currently drawn from, it would have been possible to host feasts on a very large scale. It has been estimated by Whitelaw (2001, 58) that courts 63/88, where the majority of guests were probably seated, could have held 500–800 people. In addition, the two halls 6 and 65 combined could have held a maximum of 50 more. If one accepts court 58 as an additional arena for holding guests (Bendall 2004, 124) then this figure could be raised much higher. Court 58 is open on at least one side, the south-east, hence the restrictions on space would be less, and it is *ca.* 100m^2 larger than court 63 (Bendall 2007: 92). Using Whitelaw's estimation for courts 63/88 as a guideline, possibly as many as another 1,000 could have been seated here; however, it must be stressed that his calculations are somewhat high (Bendall 2007: 91–92). The spatial analysis therefore indicates a guest list of potentially as many as 1,500 people. This is a sizeable amount and consistent with the idea of a group large enough to constitute the basis of a fighting force.

Turning to the vessels available for use, the pantry room 21 held 1,099 shallow angular bowls, a type that is suitable for eating out of (Hruby 2006, 67). This is relatively consistent with what has already been suggested. Certainly, the evidence exists for the capacity to feed approximately 1,000 guests at one time, and we would question the logic of stockpiling such large numbers of tablewares if only a small fraction was being used (though see Whitelaw 2001, 61–62).

If one examines other evidence, the scale of potential feasting provision increases further. The faunal data from various deposits in and around the palace comprise *ca.* 2 tons of meat and even a cautious analysis indicates that approximately 3,000 people may have been fed at one time (Halstead and Isaakidou 2004, 147–148). The zooarchaeological evidence is supported by the kylix count from the palace – nearly 3,000 of these drinking cups were found in the pantry room 19 alone (Hruby 2006, 52). Therefore, it appears that although only approximately 1,000 people may have actually dined in the palace's environs itself, approximately 2,000 more could have been offered hospitality of at least liquid form and/or were receiving off-cuts of meat. The number of people thus obligated to the palace through its generosity therefore increases significantly.

An obvious consideration is the fact that we have no archaeological proof that only men of an age fit for military service were guests at such feasts; indeed, the probability that women formed a proportion of the guests is very high. When examining how many people the faunal remains could have fed, however, Halstead and Isaakidou (2004, 148) intriguingly propose that the hospitality offered could have been either to a large quantity of local residents, which would obviously include women and children, or to household heads drawn from the whole polity. Using the TH Wu sealings as evidence, it appears that the administrative authority of the palace at Thebes covered an extremely large geographical area, from Mt. Helikon itself to Euboia, which was certainly not part of Thebes' territory in the Classical period (see Palaima 2004, 106). As settlements from within the whole of this area were expected on occasion to provide sacrificial animals for feasting at the palace at Thebes, might it not also be possible as well for the palace to mobilize people from such a wide area if required?

To extend this point, it appears that the palaces were taking the feasts out into the polities. On PY Vn 20, it is recorded that nine towns were provided with huge quantities of wine (410 units, estimated at 11,808 litres, Palmer 1994: 194), which has been linked with feasting events. This tablet has also been associated with Cn 608 where the same towns are instructed to fatten pigs, perhaps for the same occasion. Moreover, Hruby (2006, 70, 117) has noted the way that the vessels in the pantries at Pylos were stored could have facilitated their easy transport, thus developing the possibility that feasts were occurring regularly outside the palace (Bendall 2004, 124, 126–8). Rather than outlying settlements just receiving distributions of meat from the palaces, would it not be more effective for the palatial authority to impose its generosity on people by bringing the feast to them? The amount of obligations created would be instantly increased and the palace would have control over a larger proportion of the population in the polity. It is worth noting here that the scenes of feasting painted in hall 6 show commensality occurring *outside* (Bennet 2007, 14).

All this shows how the Mycenaeans could have recruited an army of sufficient size through feasting; it does not necessarily prove that it was the method they used. However, the great building projects and public works of the period, such as the Klytaimnestra and Atreus tholos tombs, the Cyclopean walls around Mycenae and the draining of the Copais, could only have been initiated and performed by a strong ideological motivation and/or the harnessing and exploitation of labour. As we do not have sufficient evidence for slavery on this kind of scale in the Mycenaean period, the proposal that work feasts were one method amongst others behind these building projects does seem highly likely.

Moving *corvée* labour into a more military context, Killen (2006, 73–4) has discussed the mobilization of coastguards on the Linear B tablets as a form of conscription (see also Shelmerdine 2006, 79). His reading of the PY An *o-ka* records sees these men as part-time flax workers and part-time patrol guards on the coast. As we are not proposing a Mycenaean standing army but rather the capacity to mobilize troops when required, our idea of men being called upon as necessary to serve in a military context seems to be supported by the textual evidence. It certainly appears the case in other trades such as goldsmiths and potters that *corvée* labour could be ordered by the palace (Killen 2006, 84) and there is no reason why this cannot be extended to at least part-time soldiers.

Thus far, we have concentrated in this discussion upon the wider milieu in which palatial feasts occurred and the obligations which they could create. We will now approach the issue from a different angle and examine how feasting and warfare are intertwined in ideological ways.

The Menu

Zooarchaeological evidence from the Palace of Nestor at Pylos has shown that both domesticated animals and wild game were consumed at feasts. It is not the context of serving that interests us here; rather, the hunting and killing of the wild game provides us with a metaphor for warfare and hierarchical social relations and is inextricably linked with Mycenaean feasting (Morris 1990, 149).

The social significance associated with hunting is diverse. Hunting provides an intimate link between martiality and feasting because hunting mirrors fighting while at the same time providing game to be shared with the community. In a broader spectrum, hunting embodies a number of characteristics embraced by the Mycenaean élite: predator-victim structuration mirrors social hierarchy; hunting embodies male initiation and rites of passage; and hunting embodies provision for oneself and others (Hamilakis 2003, 243–4; Morris 1990, 150). In addition, the movement through the landscape, such as that undertaken when hunting, establishes de facto ownership of the land and the game on it (Morris 1990, 150). These social aspects are important in defining the reciprocal nature of feasting that guarantees assistance in times of war.

The hunting of wild animals in its very essence is a social encounter; however the culmination of the hunt is not the termination of the social dynamic. Instead, feasting is the obvious successor to the hunting event. The feast then is not only the end of the hunt, but is also the presentation to the rest of the community of the new social status of the hunters which may have changed. In simple terms, 'the practices of feasting and drinking gave hosts and guests alike opportunities for signalling their positions and status' (Wright 2004, 50). Indeed, hunting game and sharing the meat creates a social bond between the hunter and the recipients; the hunter provides for others and receives favours in return.

Hunting is intimately tied to warfare. Besides being an arena for aggression and requiring the use of weapons, there are a number of further similarities that make hunting good preparation for battle. There are obvious parallels in the logistics of hunting and warfare: there is the handling of weapons; maintenance of physical fitness; personal bravery; tactical decision-making; stealth; and management and exploitation of the physical terrain (Morris 1990, 150). In addition, there are comparable group ideologies between hunting and conducting war, including the embodiment of maleness, designation of the other, and structuration of competitive processes and authority.

There is associated iconography connecting hunting and feasting found at Pylos. One such image, a fresco most likely positioned above hall 46, portrays men, tripods, and dogs; the dogs are hunting deer. Another fresco found in the north-west dump portrays a man holding a dead animal and a further fragment shows men carrying tripods; Wright (2004, 38–9) argues that together these compose a scene of hunting and feast preparation.

In addition to food consumption, the vast numbers of drinking vessels that have been excavated indicate that the act of drinking is central to feasting. Further evidence from the Linear B tablets record the designation of wine and meat to feasts (Piteros *et al.* 1990; Palaima 2004). There is a general correlation between drinking alcohol and aggressive behaviour. From a physiological perspective, alcohol and increased aggression are familiar bedfellows, as the alcohol blocks inhibitors in the brain and so violent tendencies are made manifest (Evans 2003; Riches 1986, 15–26). Anthropological and medical research has shown that the context of alcohol consumption dictates the behavioural expression on the part of the drinkers (Evans 2003; Riches 1986, 15–26; Wells and Graham 2003); communal drinking ceremonies have a long history on the mainland (Wright 1995; Wright 2004), and they appear to be rooted in male bonding activities. Furthermore, socializing with alcohol seems to be related to the bearing of weapons in terms of the archaeological record; weapons and drinking paraphernalia occur frequently in burials across the European Bronze Age (Sherratt 1987, 81, 89–90; Sherratt 1991; Sherratt 1994a; Sherratt 1994b; Sherratt 1995; Treherne 1995).

The ubiquity of drinking ceremonies amongst the Mycenaean élite has already been described (Wright 1995, 307); we have numerous types of archaeological evidence for wine consumption, specifically consumed in drinking rituals. There is iconographic evidence from frescoes showing men carrying wine vessels (Wright 2004, 41). We have drinking assemblages from graves, and from the palace site at Pylos. More indirect evidence comes from lists preserved in the Linear B tablets (Palmer 1995, 269), which record the production, distribution, and consumption of wine.

Contextual evidence comes from the main rooms of the Mycenaean palaces. The only frescoes portraying warfare are located in hall 64. This is situated in what has been described as the residence of the military *lawagetas*, and is adjacent to the feasting halls. Historically, there is evidence for passage into the palace past hall 64. The vignettes of active combat may be encouraging drinkers to rouse their fighting spirit (see Treherne 1995). While Bennet and Davis (1999) argue that the scenes of warfare remind visitors to the palace of how the Mycenaeans established their hegemony, it may be that the iconography of warfare portrays not just past conquests but also contemplates future scenes of domination.

The Host

There is linguistic evidence for a connection between feasting and fighting. The second-in-command in the Mycenaean palace system is the *lawagetas* and, based on the etymology of this term, *lawagetas* can be translated as *military leader* (Heubeck 1969, 173; Lindgren 1973; van Effenterre 1977; Wyatt 1994–5). The Greek word λαός is at the base of this word, and designates *troops* or *soldiers*. The word λαός does not appear in the Linear B tablets, although the *lawagetas* is often referred to. His social standing is not exactly clear: he answers to the *wanax*, the ruler, but he also controls some of the land and production of goods, seemingly independently (Palaima 1995, 129). This means the *lawagetas* has the means to sponsor large-scale feasts; that he in fact did so is recorded on the Linear B tablet PY Un 718 (Fig. 3.2).

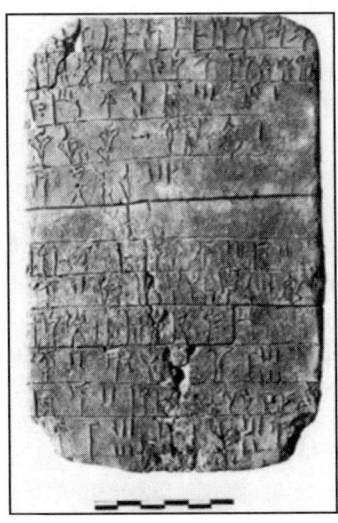

Figure 3.2. Pylos tablet Un 718 (Palaima 2004, 224). H. 19.7, W. 12.7, Th. 1.9 cm. This tablet records the lawagetas making an offering to a feast in the name of Poseidon; the military leader himself contributes to feasts. (Photograph courtesy of the photographic archives of the Program in Aegean Scripts and Prehistory, University of Texas, Austin.)

The Community

A blood sacrifice can be seen as an important aspect of feasting, as it sanctifies the communal meal (Isaakidou *et al.* 2002, 90), offers an outlet for competitive display, and enhances the feeling of common identity amongst the participants. It also stands in the liminal zone by having death support life. It is entirely possible that the Mycenaeans offered sacrifices before engaging in warfare; a sacrifice before a feast would mirror this. The parallels between sacrifice, feasting and warfare are evident; the animal nourishes the community as the fallen in battle sustain the lives of the rest of the group (Guilaine and Zammit 2005, 34).

The archaeological evidence for sacrifice is diverse. The Linear B tablets meticulously document the various benefactors of feasts and their donations. The limited range of subjects recorded on the Linear B tablets indicates the significance of this information; the benefactors are asserting their dominance by selecting and providing the victims for the sacrifice. In the iconography, the bull-procession fresco from Pylos presents us with more evidence for animal sacrifice. The scene does not show the sacrifice itself but the procession to the sacrifice, indicating that sacrifice was a communal activity (Wright 2004, 41). Other archaeological evidence for animal sacrifice includes the remains found in room 7 at Pylos. The bones were stripped off the meat before being burned in the offering; the meat was likely consumed in a feast as recorded on the Linear B tablets (Isaakidou *et al.* 2002, 88). Beside the sacrifice, a broken sword and an antique spearhead were found; while it may be conjectured that these were the instruments of sacrifice, their appearance here heightens the connection between feasting and warrior behaviour (Stocker and Davis 2004, 184).

Conclusion

While it is important to acknowledge that feasting had more than just one function, it is shown here that feasts were a natural arena in which to reinforce, compensate and celebrate martial alliances. The presence of a feasting fresco inside the main megaron underlines the relation between social power and feasting; the palace explicitly made use of the unequal nature of large-scale feasting to exact specific remuneration from their guests in the form of service. The amount of pottery and zooarchaeological evidence signifies that large groups could easily be fed, or at least plied with drink. The context of alcoholic consumption at feasts was made martial by the programme of wall paintings in hall 64, inciting drinkers to release their aggression upon state enemies, while the position of *lawagetas* as a military leader is preserved in the philology of the Linear B evidence. Moreover, hunting before feasting made use of military skills and ideology, as well as providing game. Mycenaean feasts were embedded in a complex web of social interactions that moved from hunting and social events before the feasts, to the commensality itself, to later allegiance offered to the host, creating obligations that could be fulfilled in martial situations.

References

Bennet, J. 2007. 'Representations of power in Mycenaean Pylos: script, orality, iconography', in Lang, F., Reinholdt, C. and Weilhartner, J. (eds) *ΣΤΕΦΑΝΟΣ ΑΡΙΣΤΕΙΟΣ: Archäologische Forschungen Zwischen Nil und Istros, Festschrift für Stefan Hiller zum 65. Geburtstag* (Vienna), 11–22.

Bennet, J. and Davis, J. L. 1999. 'Making Mycenaeans: warfare, territorial expansions, and representations of the other in the Pylian Kingdom', in Laffineur, R. (ed.) *POLEMOS: Le Contexte Guerrier en Egée a L'Age du Bronze, Actes de la 7e Rencontre Égéenne Internationale* (Liège), 105–20.

Bendall, L. M. 2004. 'Fit for a king? hierarchy, exclusion, aspiration and desire in the social structure of Mycenaean banqueting', in Halstead, P. and Barrett, J. C. (eds) *Food, Cuisine and Society in Prehistoric Greece* (Oxford), 105–35.

Bendall, L. M. 2007. 'How much makes a feast? accounts of banqueting foodstuffs in the Linear B records of Pylos', in Sacconi, A., Godart, L. and Negri, M. (eds) *Colloqium Romanum: Atti del XII Colloquio Internazionale di Micenologia* (Rome), 77–102.

Blegen, C. W. and Rawson, M. 1966. *The Palace of Nestor at Pylos in Western Messenia, Vol. I: The Buildings and Their Contents* (Princeton).

Deger-Jalkotzy, S. 1999. 'Military Prowess and Social Status in Mycenaean Greece', in Laffineur, R. (ed.) *POLEMOS: Le contexte guerrier en Egée a l'age du bronze, actes de la 7e rencontre égéenne internationale* (Liège: Université de Liège), 121–31.

Dietler, M. 2001. 'Theorizing the Feast: Rituals of Consumption, Commensal Politics, and Power in African Contexts', in Dietler, M. and Hayden, B. (eds) *Feasts: Archaeological and Ethnographic Perspectives on Food, Politics and Power* (Washington: Smithsonian Institution Press), 65–114.

Dietler, M. and Herbich, I. 2001. 'Feasts and labor mobilization: dissecting a fundamental economic practice', in Dietler, M. and Hayden, B. (eds) *Feasts: Archaeological and Ethnographic Perspectives on Food, Politics and Power* (Washington), 240–64.

Evans, C. M. 2003. 'Alcohol, violence and aggression', *Alcohol and Alcoholism* **15.3**, 104–117.

Guilaine, J. and Zammit, J. 2005. *The Origins of War: Violence in Prehistory* (Oxford).

Halstead, P. and Isaakidou, V. 2004. 'Faunal evidence for feasting: burnt offerings from the Palace of Nestor at Pylos', in Halstead, P. and Barrett, J. C. (eds) *Food, Cuisine and Society in Prehistoric Greece* (Oxford), 136–54.

Hamilakis, Y. 2003. 'The sacred geography of hunting: wild animals, social power and gender in early farming societies', in Kotjabopoulou, E., Hamilakis, Y., Halstead, P., Gamble, C. and Elefanti, P. (eds) *Zooarchaeology in Greece: Recent Advances* (London), 239–47.

Heubeck, A. 1969. 'Gedanken zu griech. laos', in *Studi Linguistici in onore di Vittore Pisani* (Brescia), 535–44.

Hruby, J. A. 2006. *Feasting and Ceramics: a View from the Palace of Nestor at Pylos*. Unpublished PhD dissertation, University of Cincinnati.

Isaakidou, V., Halstead, P., Davis, J. L. and Stocker, S. 2002. 'Burnt animal sacrifice at the Mycenaean 'Palace of Nestor', Pylos', *Antiquity* **76**, 86–92.

Killen, J. T. 2006. 'Conscription and corvée at Mycenaean Pylos', in Perna, M. (ed.) *Fiscality in Mycenaean and Near Eastern Archives* (Paris), 73–87.

Lemonnier, P. 1996. 'Food, competition, and the status of food in New Guinea', in Wiessner, P. and Schiefenhövel, W. (eds) *Food and the Status Quest: An Interdisciplinary Perspective* (Oxford), 219–34.

Lindgren, M. 1973. *The People of Pylos: Prosopographical and Methodological Studies in the Pylos Archives* (Uppsala).

Morris, C. 1990. 'In pursuit of the white tusked boar', in Hägg, R. and Nordquist, G. (eds) *Celebrations of Death and Divinity in the Bronze Age Argolid: Proceedings of the Sixth International Symposium at the Swedish Institute at Athens, 11–13 June, 1988* (Stockholm), 149–56.

Palaima, T. G. 1995. 'The nature of the Mycenaean *Wanax*: non-Indo-European origins and priestly functions', in Rehak, P. (ed.) *The Role of the Ruler in the Prehistoric Aegean: Proceedings of a Panel Discussion*

Presented at the Annual Meeting of the Archaeological Institute of America, New Orleans, Louisiana, 28 December 1992 (Liège: Université de Liège), 119–42.

Palaima, T. G. 2004. 'Sacrificial feasting in the Linear B tablets', in Wright, J. C. (ed.) *The Mycenaean Feast* (Princeton), 97–126.

Palmer, R. 1994. *Wine in the Mycenaean Palace Economy [Aegaeum 10]* (Liège).

Palmer, R. 1995. 'Wine and viticulture in the Linear A and B texts of the Bronze Age Aegean', in McGovern, P. E., Fleming, S. J. and Katz, S. H. (eds) *The Origins and Ancient History of Wine: Food and Nutrition in History and Anthropology* (Philadelphia), 269–85.

Perodie, J.R. 2001. 'Feasting for prosperity: a study of southern northwest coast feasting', in Dietler, M. and Hayden, B. (eds) *Feasts: Archaeological and Ethnographic Perspectives on Food, Politics, and Power* (Washington), 185–214.

Piteros, C., Olivier, J.-P. and Melena, J. L. 1990. 'Les inscriptions en Linéaire B des nodules de Thèbes (1982): la fouille, les documents, les possibilités d'interprétation', *Bulletin de Correspondance Hellénique* **114**, 103–184.

Riches, D. 1986. 'The phenomenon of violence', in Riches, D. (ed.) *The Anthropology of Violence* (Oxford) 1–27.

Shelmerdine, C. W. 2006. 'Mycenaean palatial administration', in Deger-Jalkotzy, S. and Lemos, I. S. (eds) *Ancient Greece: From the Mycenaean Palaces to the Age of Homer* (Edinburgh), 73–86.

Sherratt, A. 1987. 'Cups that cheered: the introduction of alcohol to Prehistoric Europe', in Waldren, W. and Kennard, R. C. (eds) *Bell Beakers of the Western Mediterranean* (Oxford), 81–114.

Sherratt, A. 1991. 'Sacred and profane substances: the ritual use of narcotics in Later Neolithic Europe', in Garwood, P., Jennings D., Skeates, R. and Toms, J. (eds) *Sacred and Profane: Proceedings of a Conference on Archaeology, Ritual and Religion, Oxford 1989* (Oxford), 50–64.

Sherratt, A. 1994a. 'Core, periphery and margin: perspectives on the Bronze Age', in Mathers, C. and Stoddart, S. (eds) *Development and Decline in the Mediterranean Bronze Age* (Sheffield), 335–46.

Sherratt, A. 1994b. 'The emergence of élites: Earlier Bronze Age Europe, 2500–1300 BC', in Cunliffe, B. (ed.) *The Oxford Illustrated Prehistory of Europe* (Oxford), 244–76.

Sherratt, A. 1995. 'Alcohol and its alternatives: symbol and substance in pre-industrial cultures', in Goodman, J., Lovejoy, P. E. and Sherratt, A. (eds) *Consuming Habits: Drugs in History and Anthropology* (London), 11–47.

Stocker, S. and Davis, J. L. 2004. 'Animal sacrifice, archives, and feasting at the Palace of Nestor', in Wright, J. C. (ed.) *The Mycenaean Feast* (Princeton), 59–75.

Treherne, P. 1995. 'The warrior's beauty: the masculine body and self-identity in Bronze-Age Europe', *Journal of European Archaeology* **3** (1), 105–44.

Van Effenterre, H. 1977. 'Laos, laoi et lawagetas', *Kadmos* **16** (1), 36–55.

Wells, S. and Graham, K. 2003. 'Aggression involving alcohol: relationship to drinking patterns and social context', *Addiction* **98** (1), 33–42.

Whitelaw, T. 2001. 'Reading between the tablets: assessing Mycenaean palatial involvement in ceramic production and consumption', in Voutsaki, S. and Killen, J. (eds) *Economy and Politics in the Mycenaean Palace States: Proceedings of a Conference Held on 1–3 July 1999 in the Faculty of Classics, Cambridge* (Cambridge), 51–79.

Wiessner, P. 2001. 'Of feasting and value: Enga feasts in a historical perspective (Papua New Guinea)', in Dietler, M. and Hayden, B. (eds) *Feasts: Archaeological and Ethnographic Perspectives on Food, Politics and Power* (Washington), 115–43.

Wright, J. C. 1995. 'Empty cups and empty jugs: the social role of wine in Minoan and Mycenaean societies', in McGovern, P. E., Fleming, S. J. and Katz, S. H. (eds) *The Origins and Ancient History of Wine: Food and Nutrition in History and Anthropology* (Philadelphia), 287–307.

Wright, J. C. 2004. 'A survey of evidence for feasting in Mycenaean society', in Wright, J. C. (ed.) *The Mycenaean Feast* (Princeton), 13–58.

Wyatt, W. 1994–5. 'Homeric and Mycenaean Laos', *Minos* **29–30**, 159–70.

'The Privilege of Civilization':
Cultural Change at the Victorian Dining Table

Annie Gray,
University of York

Introduction

This paper is situated within the field of historical archaeology: the archaeology of the recent past (here taken to mean after *ca.* 1600). As such, it uses the full range of data available to the historical archaeologist – documentary and material – but places these within a set of paradigms and theoretical approaches that are explicitly archaeological. It does this by considering how food was consumed in the Victorian period – focusing on the dining practices of the middle and upper classes – as opposed to how food was produced or distributed. It is hoped that the conclusions reached will not only be of benefit to historical archaeology, but will also contribute to the wider historical and culinary historical context.

The 'Georgian Order'

To date few studies specifically on food and dining have been carried out within historical archaeology. One exception is James Deetz's (1996) influential publication *In Small Things Forgotten* which demonstrated, to a popular as well as academic audience, how everyday objects can inform on the lives of often neglected social groups (Brooks 2000, 16–17). His work influenced not only mainstream historical archaeological thinking, but also the neo-Marxist school exemplified by Shackel (1993). Deetz (1996) concentrated on the period up to *ca.* 1800 and drew upon foodways and their associated material culture to illustrate the application of the theory of a 'Georgian Order'. His work was founded upon Glassie's (1975) analysis of folk housing which attempted to describe underlying structures and patterns as a reflection of contemporary mentalities, but acknowledges the place of individual human action in perpetuating and/or challenging those mentalities.

Recent work continues to emphasize the role of the individual at the centre of cultural change (Johnson 1996; Leone 2005). Examination of the concept of individuality has drawn upon evidence from faunal remains, ceramics and documentary sources to indicate the physical separation of diners and the regulation of their portions in the nineteenth century (Fitts 1999). Shackel (1993) uses the example of forks, and other objects, to suggest a link between dining and bodily self-control as part of a process which imposed discipline, not just on the self, but also on others through the medium

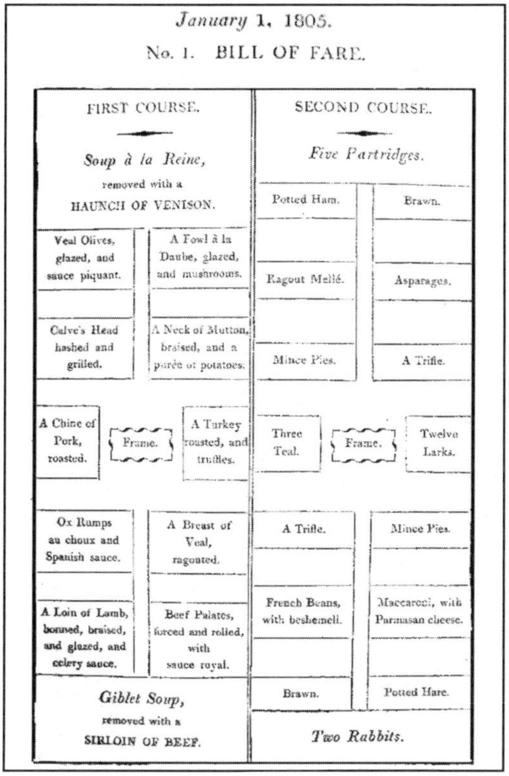
January 1, 1805.

No. 1. BILL OF FARE.

FIRST COURSE.			SECOND COURSE.		
Soup à la Reine, removed with a HAUNCH OF VENISON.			*Five Partridges.*		
			Potted Ham.		Brawn.
Veal Olives, glazed, and sauce piquant.		A Fowl à la Daube, glazed, and mushrooms.	Ragout Mellé.		Asparagus.
Calve's Head hashed and grilled.		A Neck of Mutton, braised, and a purée of potatoes.	Mince Pies.		A Trifle.
A Chine of Pork, roasted.	Frame.	A Turkey roasted, and truffles.	Three Teal.	Frame.	Twelve Larks.
Ox Rumps au choux and Spanish sauce.		A Breast of Veal, ragouted.	A Trifle.		Mince Pies.
A Loin of Lamb, bonned, braised, and glazed, and celery sauce.		Beef Palates, forced and rolled, with sauce royal.	French Beans, with beshemeli.		Maccaroni, with Parmasan cheese.
			Brawn.		Potted Hare.
Giblet Soup, removed with a SIRLOIN OF BEEF.			*Two Rabbits.*		

Figure 4.1. Service à la Française. *(Simpson 1807, courtesy of the Brotherton Library, Leeds). Photograph by A. Gray.*

of material culture. The idea that the Victorian period saw an increased emphasis on the individual is also suggested by wider shifts in serving styles, which it is important to consider in more detail.

The Dynamics of Serving Styles

By the late eighteenth century the form of dining that Elias (1939) regards as the epitome of civilization had developed, as shown in figure 4.1. According to cookbooks and visual depictions, service *à la Française* (known in America as 'Old English' (DiZerega Wall 1994)) consisted of three or four courses with all the dishes in each course presented on the table at the same time (Brears 1994). Each course moved, in general, from heavy to light, and the meal culminated in dessert. Dishes were laid out symmetrically, sometimes using tablecloth folds or the indentations left by previous courses as guides (Cosnett 1825). Servants were on hand to serve drinks from the sideboard and to clear and replenish the table (Brown 1990). On the surface, *à la Française* seems to be communal and potentially riotous; however, an elaborate system of etiquette surrounded it, both for servants and guests (for further details see Paston-Williams 1993; Brears 1994). Those who made mistakes could find themselves not only

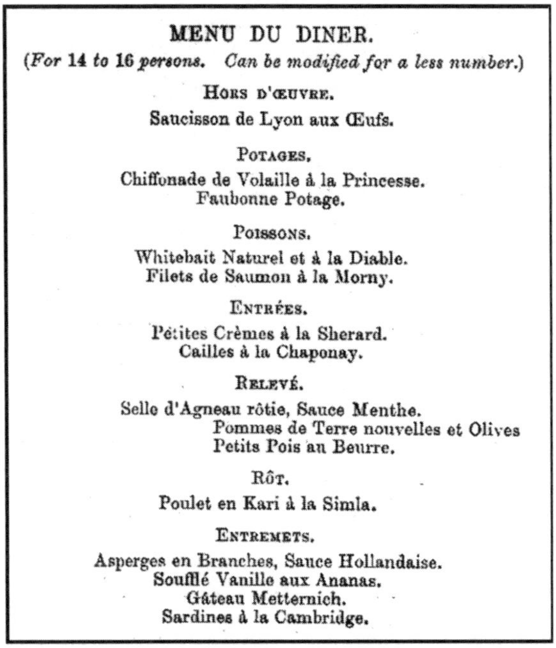

> **MENU DU DINER.**
> *(For 14 to 16 persons. Can be modified for a less number.)*
>
> HORS D'ŒUVRE.
> Saucisson de Lyon aux Œufs.
>
> POTAGES.
> Chiffonade de Volaille à la Princesse.
> Faubonne Potage.
>
> POISSONS.
> Whitebait Naturel et à la Diable.
> Filets de Saumon à la Morny.
>
> ENTRÉES.
> Pétites Crèmes à la Sherard.
> Cailles à la Chaponay.
>
> RELEVÉ.
> Selle d'Agneau rôtie, Sauce Menthe.
> Pommes de Terre nouvelles et Olives
> Petits Pois au Beurre.
>
> RÔT.
> Poulet en Kari à la Simla.
>
> ENTREMETS.
> Asperges en Branches, Sauce Hollandaise.
> Soufflé Vanille aux Ananas.
> Gâteau Metternich.
> Sardines à la Cambridge.

Figure 4.2. Service à la Russe. *(Marshall* ca. *1888). Photograph by A. Gray.*

socially embarrassed, but also professionally disadvantaged (Brown 1990, 14). With no imposed limits, self-control was key, and seen as a means of differentiating the civilized being from the savage – crucial at a time when debate raged on the nature of men versus women versus untamed nature (Clery 2004). The nature of *à la Française* lent itself to gratuitous display, but within that could be demonstrated refined restraint. George IV, certainly not the best example of self-discipline, nevertheless demonstrated his civilized credentials at his Coronation Feast in 1822, when he sampled just four of the 20 dishes on offer in one course (Day 2000, 50).

Between the 1810s and 1890s service *à la Française* was gradually replaced by a more linear type of service – *à la Russe* (Mars 1994). Dinner services in collections, inventories and sales catalogues, as well as evidence from menus, indicate that the new style was commonplace among the middle and upper classes by the end of the nineteenth century, although the survival of earlier styles under new names – supper and high tea – indicates that the guidelines laid down in advice books were not whole-heartedly accepted. As shown in figure 4.2, the new service style consisted of more courses but normally with a choice of only two or three dishes in each. Portions were allotted in the kitchen or, in one variation designed to incorporate the display of an English roast, at the sideboard. A significant characteristic of *à la Russe* was the illusion of privileging the individual, the importance of this concept can be seen in the portioned mutton cutlets, small moulded ices and filleted meats and fish. However, compared to the freedom of *à la Française* this service style actually meant the decline of individuality because choice was curtailed in favour of imposed uniformity (Kaufman 2002).

Cultural Change at the Victorian Dining Table

Initially *à la Russe* appears more expensive than *à la Française* due to the number of servants required and because it attempts to exclude social inferiors. Based on the evidence of cookbooks, *à la Russe* does seem to have been adopted by the wealthy at first (Jameson 1987). However, cookbooks for the upper classes tended to be written by known chefs (e.g. Francatelli and Soyer), who would naturally promote a new style that favoured the professionalization of cookery (Kaufman 2002). Yet viewed from a middle-class perspective, *à la Russe* has more to offer in many ways than its predecessor. Certain authors, for instance Jewry (*ca.* 1878), asserted that *à la Russe* was cheaper and therefore better suited to her middle-class readership – provided they knew what to do, which, thanks to the flourishing self-help market, they would.

On the Table

By the end of the nineteenth century, a typical table was divided down the middle with flowers and other decorations, emphasizing the vertical plane, in a determined move away from the shared intimacy of *à la Française*. From a conversational viewpoint, a guest's dinner companions would be limited to their immediate neighbours. Correct placement of diners in order to optimize sociability was paramount, and through this a hostess' knowledge of her guests could be judged. With *à la Russe*, everything had to be at hand, and preferably not shared. Jameson (1987) attributes this to a growing fastidiousness and concern over hygiene, which can be seen in other areas of society. It also reflects notions of property – for the duration of the dinner, the diner 'owned' their place setting. This is one reason for the proliferation of objects associated with nineteenth-century dining.

As a tool for display, service *à la Française* necessitated a range of plates and serving vessels. Dessert services were especially flamboyant, designed to reflect candlelight at the end of a satisfying meal. Despite archaeological concern with the idea of matching sets (DiZerega Wall 1994, 144), evidence suggests a more nuanced approach to ceramic dining ware. At Harewood House, Yorkshire, three distinct sets of dining ware of overlapping periods exist, complementing each other, but not matching. Eighteenth-century Coalport dessert ware shows clear signs of sustained use, including a number of plates converted into tazzes in the mid-nineteenth century. This may be an example of the importance of patina, or indicate that some data are missing from the site-derived record. The cost of fitting out a large table for *à la Française* could be huge, and some hosts, at least, preferred to rent. Harewood probably rented a gold dinner service for the visit of Queen Victoria in 1835 (Gallimore pers. comm.).

The amount of dining equipment available by the end of the nineteenth century was phenomenal: asparagus servers, grape spoons and a whole array of tools for fish are evident in any household goods catalogue (Bosomworth 1991). While this looks like increasing the cost of dinners and certainly spurred on manufacturers, it is deceptive. With *à la Russe*, a large array of different plates was no longer required: small, affordable objects could be purchased instead, along with increasingly plain tableware. Not everything had to be bought immediately. Indeed, it would be easy for a family starting out to follow Jewry's (*ca.* 1878) advice and host dinner parties in May – asparagus season – based on an investment in asparagus equipment and little else other than fresh flowers. Archaeological investigation suggests that flowers formed part of the repertoire of middle-class households in Britain and its wider sphere of influence (Fitts 1999; Young 2003), suggesting that they followed the guidelines of the advice books. Specialist tools could be exclusive if the knowledge of how to use them was lacking, but information was readily available in books and manuals, provided the aspiring diner was prepared to invest time and money in keeping up-to-date. If, as Emerson (1856) suggested, 'not the Trial by Jury, but the dinner is the capital institution,' it was better, surely, for those not bred into its intricacies, to encourage such trial by methods which could be learnt, than to risk the more fluid, open structure of service *à la Française*.

Ceramic Design

A brief consideration of the design of tableware also suggests that middle-class requirements may have played a greater role in the changing nature of English dining than previously recognized. While bearing in mind the range of living standards and attitudes encompassed by the term 'middle class', it is possible to consider the identity of this self-aware and, to a large extent, self-constructed group through the material culture they consumed. More work needs to be undertaken on class structure and examining patterns of purchase, but as Brooks (1999) has demonstrated, even broad-scale investigations of ceramic design can yield significant results. For instance, visual trends in the nineteenth century show a move from the exotic/oriental, through romantic English, to natural, often botanical, designs, and finally to neutral or abstract forms.

The decline of the oriental was in part due to the cessation of porcelain imports by the East India Company (Goss 2005, 14), and subsequent spur to British manufactures. As Brooks (1999) argues, it also reflects growing national sentiment. Both the bucolic landscapes of the second quarter of the nineteenth century, and the naturalistic yet decontextualized botanicals of the third indicate the masking of social stresses by everyday symbolism (Young 2003). The latter also suggests a link to the growth of suburbia and a harking back to a less industrialized age. Gothic designs occur at a similar time. American studies have linked the popularity of the gothic to the cult of domesticity and accompanying religious revival (Clark 1988). While less of a force in England itself, such concepts certainly played a role in influencing consumer choices: Queen Victoria, who deliberately publicized her role as wife and mother alongside that of Head of State, possessed at least one gothic tea service (OH 1901, unpublished). The abstract patterns of the late nineteenth century not only take the decontextualization of modern life further, but at the same time show the markedly militaristic bent of society. These trends occur, not only at the dinner table, but also on teawares and other ceramics, indicating the degree to which underlying attitudes permeated everyday Victorian life.

Enforcing Status: Food and the Written Word

Inevitably much of the archaeological work on eighteenth- and nineteenth-century dining draws heavily upon written evidence, both as a source of data but also to provide a wider context for interpretation (for instance Jameson 1987). Documentary evidence is as much a creation of past societies as the artefacts that are the accepted concern of archaeologists and should be regarded in the same way: as active agents in the creation and negotiation of personal and group identities (Fitts 1999, 39–40; Moreland 2001). Evidence from etiquette and cookbooks should not therefore be either accepted or disregarded unthinkingly, but rather studied as a whole using an archaeological approach to consider factors other than just the information contained in the words. This section demonstrates the way in which texts can be used as artefacts to enhance wider understanding of the way in which the mentality of *à la Russe* was used to control and regulate the Victorian household.

Figure 4.3 shows a spread from a provisioning ledger for Osborne House, Isle of Wight. The various groups of people to be fed, together with their allotted meals, are laid out in status order across the pages. Queen Victoria's table (lunch and dinner) occupies the primary position at the far left, while on the right-hand page can be found the Steward's Room, the electricians, choristers, nurses, sick room, police and so forth. The Governess's ambivalent position is illustrated in the way in which her section drifts from page to page throughout the ledger. A comparison of the Queen's and the household's dinner elucidates Queen Victoria's domestic arrangements at Osborne in the last years of her life.

The phenomenal amount of food available at the table is an indication not only of largesse, but also of the Queen's renowned appetite (Hunter pers. comm.). *À la Russe* service ensured that portions would be tailored, but it was still possible to eat what Paston-Williams (1993, 254) calls a 'suicidally large diet'. Throughout the ledger, dishes are written in French unless they were of German origin or offered from the sideboard, which tended to hold traditional English fare such as roast beef and, at Christmas, boar's head. By 1897, this style of service was considered old-fashioned, perhaps a reflection of the Queen's tastes at the age of 78, or perhaps a means of proclaiming her Englishness above her fashion sense. In contrast, the Household Dinner is *à la Russe* in its most elaborate form. The Queen made it clear that Osborne was a retreat from the formality of court life in London and perceived herself as living a 'normal' life (Hunter, pers.comm). This difference in styles is one indication that she was attempting a lower-key existence than that of her attendants. It also highlights the problem of reliance on etiquette books as a source: it must be remembered that they are aspirational, and generalize about social practice.

At the next social level down – the Steward's Room – menus are written in English, and the layout is more ambiguous, ceasing to divide courses rigidly, and indicating that for most of the groups fed at Osborne changing service styles had little impact upon the table (Fig. 4.3). The categorizations in the ledger again give the illusion of

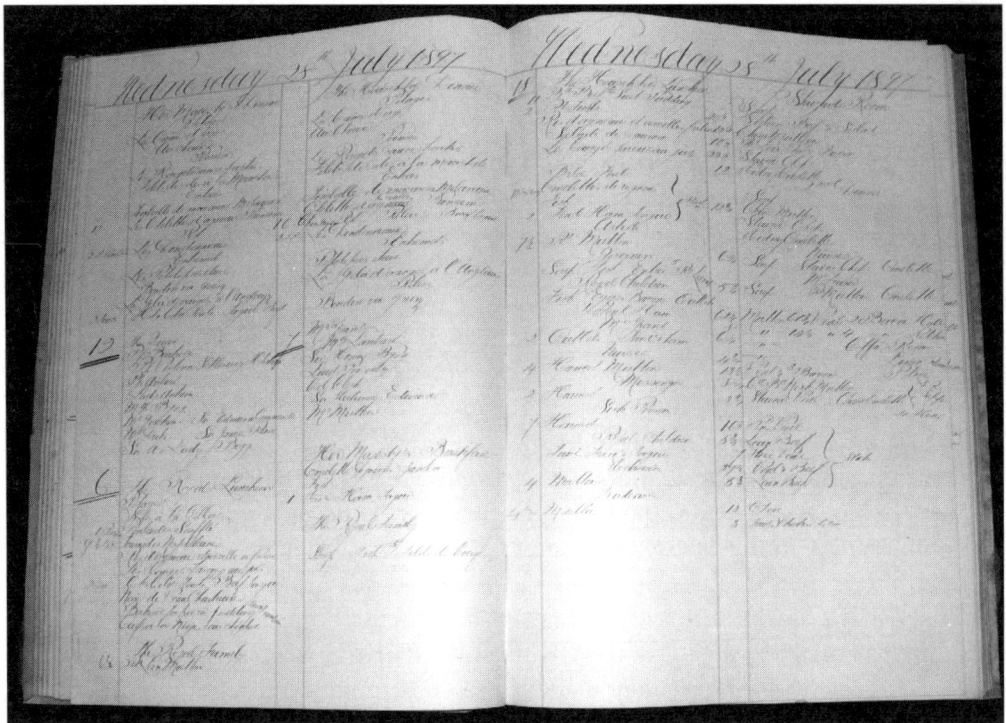

Figure 4.3. Osborne House provisioning ledger entry for July 28th, 1897. Courtesy of Osborne House (English Heritage). Photograph by A. Gray. Below, a transcript of the ledger.

The Queen's Dinner (12 people)	The Household Dinner (7 people)
Potages	Potages
La Crème d'Orgue	*La Crème d'Orgue*
Au Choux	*Au Choux*
Poissons	Poissons
Les Rougets Sauce Hachis	*Les Rougets Sauce Hachis*
Filets de Soles à la Maréchale	*Filets de Soles à la Maréchale*
Rôt	Rôt
Les Dindonneaux	*Les Dindonneaux*
Entrées	Entrées
Timbale de Macaroni Milanese	*Timbale de Macaroni Milanese*
Les Cotelettes d'Agneau Princesse	*Les Cotelettes d'Agneau Princesse*
Entremêts	Réleve
Les Pois Etuvé	*Boeuf Braisé*
Boudin von Griesz	
La Gelee d'Orange a l'Anglaise	Entremêts
	Les Pois Etuvé
Sideboard	*La Gelee d'Orange a l'Anglaise*
Hot & Cold Fowls	
Tongue	Réleve
Beef	*Boudin von Griesz*

increasing awareness of the individual, dividing the household into ever smaller groups. However, names are noted only for the two top tables and, where specific, high-ranking individuals require special meals such as travelling baskets. The Governess is never named although a Mr Frazer features frequently. He was probably one of the Highland servants (Hunter pers. comm.) and, as such, outside the norms of aristocratic household division. At the other extreme, the lower servants are denoted only by the place in which they eat ('hall', 'coffee room' and so on). The individual is, therefore, entirely missing from this household *à la Russe*, which, in its rigid application of internal hierarchy even in a working document of this type, reflects the way in which the Victorian mentality had embraced the dictatorial, highly formal style of *à la Russe*, and implemented it as a global domestic system.

Conclusion

This paper has provided an example of the way in which archaeological methodologies and theories can be applied to dining culture in nineteenth century Britain. The period is a significant one in the development of the modern world. Victorian Britain struggled to come to terms with the rapid changes occasioned by industrialization, social mobility, war and the commodification of culture. Even a brief consideration of dining in the period yields valuable evidence of the way in which strategies were implemented to cope with these tensions. It furthermore suggests that most of these strategies were invented by the middle and upper middle classes, and that, far from adhering to a straightforward centrist or emulative model, changes were complex and very gradual. The decline of individual power and the constraint of personal choice were effectively disguised by the new stress placed on personal property, as reflected in place settings and service styles. As I have suggested, many individuals became objects, to be moved around and slotted into formulas at will; perhaps in this we see the birth of the modern world.

Acknowledgements

This paper is based on PhD research made possible by an AHRC studentship. Thanks are due to Michael Hunter, Curator at Osborne House, for allowing me access to the archives and giving generously both time and advice. Thanks also to Melissa Gallimore of Harewood House and to an anonymous referee for commenting upon a previous draft.

References

MANUSCRIPT SOURCES

OH (1901, unpublished) Osborne House Inventory.

PRINTED SOURCES

Bosomworth, D. 1991. *The Victorian Catalogue of Household Goods* (London).

Brears, P. 1994. 'A la Française: the waning of a long dining tradition', in Wilson, C. A. (ed.) *Luncheon, Nuncheon and Other Meals: Eating with the Victorians* (Stroud), 91–116.

Brooks, A. 1999. 'Building Jerusalem: transfer printed finewares and the creation of British identity', in Tarlow, S. and West, S. (ed.) *The Familiar Past? Archaeologies of Later Historical Britain* (London), 51–65.

Brooks, A. 2000. *The Comparative Analysis of Late Eighteenth and Nineteenth Century Ceramics – A Transatlantic Perspective* (University of York).

Brown, P. 1990. *Pyramids of Pleasure: Eating and Dining in the Eighteenth Century* (York).

Clark, C. 1988. 'Domestic architecture as an index to social history: the romantic revival and the cult of domesticity in America, 1840–1870', in George, R. B. S. (ed.) *Material Life in Ameria, 1600–1860* (Boston), 535–542.

Clery, E. 2004. *The Feminisation Debate in Eighteenth Century England: Literature, Commerce and Luxury* (Basingstoke).

Cosnett, T. 1825. *The Footman's Directory* (London).

Day, I. 2000. *Eat, Drink and be Merry* (London).

Deetz, J. 1996. *In Small Things Forgotten: An Archaeology of Early American Life* (New York).

DiZerega Wall, D. 1994. *The Archaeology of Gender: Separating the Spheres in Urban America* (New York).

Elias, N. 1939. *The Civilising Process* (Oxford).

Emerson, R. 1856. "English Traits." Retrieved June, 2007, from http://www.emersoncentral.com/manners_english.htm.

Fitts, R. 1999. 'The archaeology of middle-class domesticity and gentility in Victorian Brooklyn', *Historical Archaeology* **33**(1), 39–62.

Glassie, H. 1975. *Folk Housing in Middle Virginia* (Knoxville).

Goss, S. 2005. *British Teapots and Coffee Pots* (Princes Risborough).

Jameson, R. 1987. 'Purity and power at the Victorian dinner party', in Hodder, I. (ed.) *The Archaeology of Contextual Meanings* (Cambridge), 55–65.

Jewry, M. *ca.* 1878. *Warne's Everyday Cookery* (London).

Johnson, M. 1996. *An Archaeology of Capitalism* (Oxford).

Kaufman, C. 2002. 'Structuring the meal: the revolution of Service à la Russe', in Walker, H. (ed.) *The Meal: Proceedings of the Oxford Symposium on Food and Cookery, 2001* (Totnes), 123–133.

Leone, M. 2005. *The Archaeology of Liberty in an American Capital: Excavations in Annapolis* (Berkeley).

Mars, V. 1994. 'A La Russe: the new way of dining', in Wilson, C. A. (ed.) *Luncheon, Nuncheon and Other Meals: Eating with the Victorans* (Stroud), 117–144.

Moreland, J. 2001. *Archaeology and Text* (London).

Paston-Williams, S. 1993. *The Art of Dining: A History of Cooking and Eating* (London).

Shackel, P. 1993. *Personal Discipline and Material Culture: An Archaeology of Annapolis, Maryland, 1695–1870* (Knoxville).

Young, L. 2003. *Middle Class Culture in the Nineteenth Century: America, Australia, Britain* (Basingstoke).

Take it with a Pinch of Salt?
Thinking about the Cultural Significance of Producing and Consuming Salt

*Sarah-Jane Hathaway,
University of Bournemouth*

Introduction

This paper is the result of my ongoing doctoral research into the archaeological evidence for prehistoric and Romano-British coastal salt production in southern Britain. The main aims of this research are to assess the current knowledge on this subject, explore new sites and offer further insights into the significance of salt production. It is becoming clear that not only do we need to readdress the recording and interpretation of the archaeological evidence itself, we also need to incorporate the cultural significance of producing and consuming salt in the past. This includes the use of salt to preserve food, as well as the issue of taste. Salt is not the same the world over; the size of the crystals and its taste are dependent on the location, time and the methods used to extract it. The look of salt is also variable; it is not always white but can include a spectrum of reds, pinks and greys. I am exploring the role of salt all over the world, within prehistory and history, considering ethnographic evidence and customs, traditions and superstitions that are still embedded within our culture today. Examining this subject area with an open and holistic approach is key to expanding our knowledge of past societies.

Salt Production

Salt has played an important role throughout human history, and humans have chosen to actively produce it for thousands of years. This could have been for reasons of need, want, or both. We need salt to live, but at some point the *need* for salt presumably grew to include *want*. New research has located salt production-sites that date to the Neolithic period in Romania (Chapman *et al.* 2001), with further Bronze Age sites located across Europe (Nenquin 1961). In Britain, there is evidence that salt has been produced from the sea for at least 3000 years, with the majority of known salt production-sites dating to the Late Iron Age and early Romano-British period. Many of these sites are distributed across the Somerset Levels (Grove and Brunning 1998; Leech 1981; Rippon 2000), stretching around the coast to Essex (Fawn *et al.* 1990; Nenquin 1961) and Lincolnshire (Chowne 2001; Lane and Morris 2001).

Archaeological evidence for salt production in the prehistoric and Romano-British period comprises a variety of associated features and material commonly known as

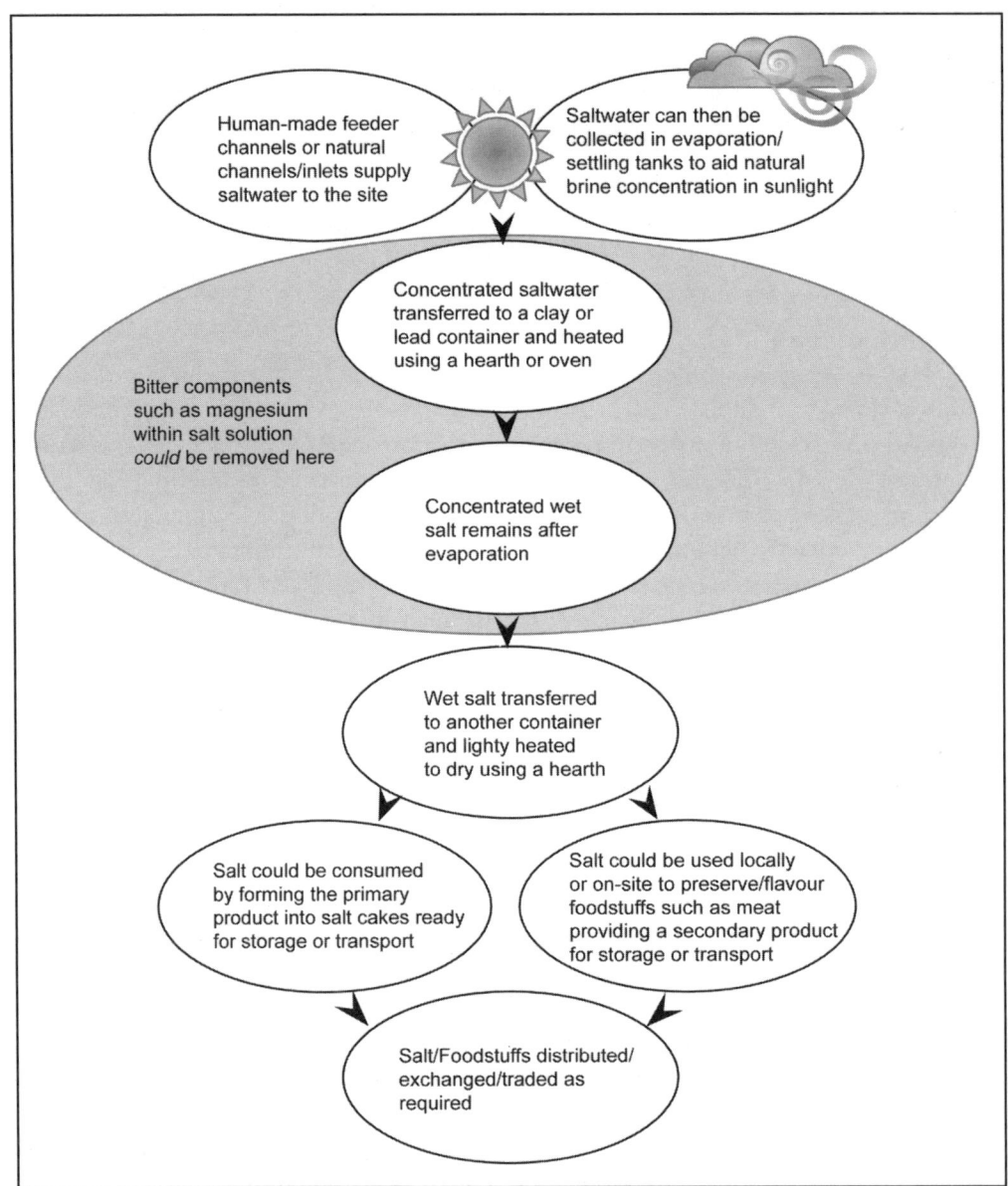

Figure 5.1. Diagram showing a method of coastal salt production.

'briquetage'. Briquetage is the generic term for the ceramic equipment used on-site to produce salt. Its form varies from site to site but usually consists of containers and their supports, as well as general hearth lining and furniture. This material is often overlooked, but the discovery of it in coastal areas is traditionally used to define the presence of salt production-sites. The associated features are less well understood and are in great need of further analysis, something this research aims to achieve. Work by Lane and Morris (2001) has begun to address the issue. They have identified the features as working areas, ovens, enclosed hearths, open hearths, water management features (such as settling tanks and channels supplying water) and general debris deposition areas, including mounds. On the basis of these interpretations it is possible to reconstruct, albeit simplistically, the methods by which salt was produced during prehistory and the Romano-British period (see Fig. 5.1). Beyond understanding the technology of salt production, the cultural significance of its consumption is also in need of analysis.

Salt Consumption

Here the term 'consumption' includes the consumption of production-site, the briquetage as well as the salt itself.

Site consumption incorporates the series of human actions performed in order to produce salt. An understanding of this performance can be gleaned by examining the visual relationship between features on archaeological production-sites and by considering, through experimental archaeology, how specific tasks took place within the given space. Salt production-sites are frequently viewed as 'functional', regarded as representing an almost abstract seasonal 'process' that took place on the periphery of everyday life and required little effort or skill. Having personally taken part in archaeological experiments to produce salt using traditional methods, it is clear that this conventional interpretation is invalid: much time and effort is required, from the 'pre-production' preparation to the production itself. Salt production, and the use of space it involves, is as complex as any other production activity, such as pottery manufacture.

Investigation of briquetage consumption requires the analysis of assemblages from both within and outside production-sites. The potential of briquetage to tell us about human choices in the past has often been underestimated and its lifecycle – how it was treated and used during and after salt production – is in need of further exploration. Figure 5.2 presents a simple lifecycle of briquetage. The first part of the sequence is associated with its creation and primary consumption, the second and third parts involve its distribution, secondary consumption and subsequent deposition.

Briquetage has been found inland at hillforts and settlement sites, and is thought to have been used to transport salt from the coast (Morris 1994). It has also been re-cycled, as at Ower, Poole Harbour, where it was used to create a working floor (Sunter and Woodward 1987). There are two early Romano-British examples – from Burradon, Tyne and Wear, and Melsonby, North Yorkshire – where briquetage was apparently deposited deliberately in the terminals of Romano-British hut gullies (Willis 1999). At Burradon, two pits were placed within a filled eavesdrop gully associated with a large circular structure. According to Willis (1999, 96) they were 'about the most artefact rich deposits' within the site, producing fragments of pottery, briquetage and Dressel 20 amphora. The situation at Melsonby was very similar; pits containing briquetage and Dressel 20 amphora being cut into an eavesdrop gully and an associated ditch. The

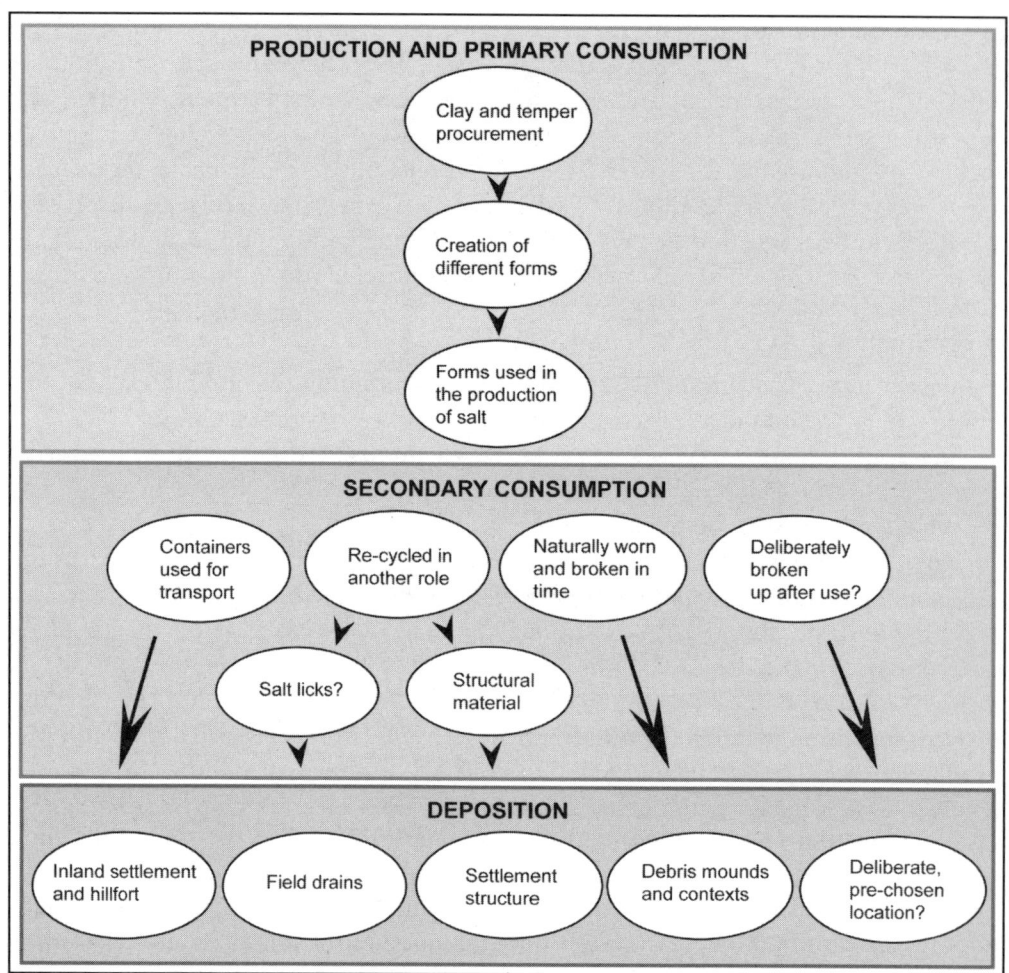

Figure 5.2. The lifecycle of briquetage.

general scarcity of pits on these two sites, together with a wider dearth of briquetage and amphora in the regions led Willis to interpret the deposition of briquetage as symbolic. He concluded that the deposition of everyday and exotic goods at the end of occupation constitutes a final act 'bound up with acts of recall or acknowledgement of what had gone before' (Willis 1999, 99).

Most briquetage deposition, however, occurred on or close to salt production-sites. Thousands of fragments are found in 'waste' mounds, as at the famous Red Hill mounds of Essex (De Brisay 1975). It has been suggested that the fragmentary nature of briquetage, specifically found within the actual boundaries of the site, could represent deliberate breakage of briquetage as a final act, representing the completion of the production event (De Brisay 1978). Perhaps this act took place at the end of each season

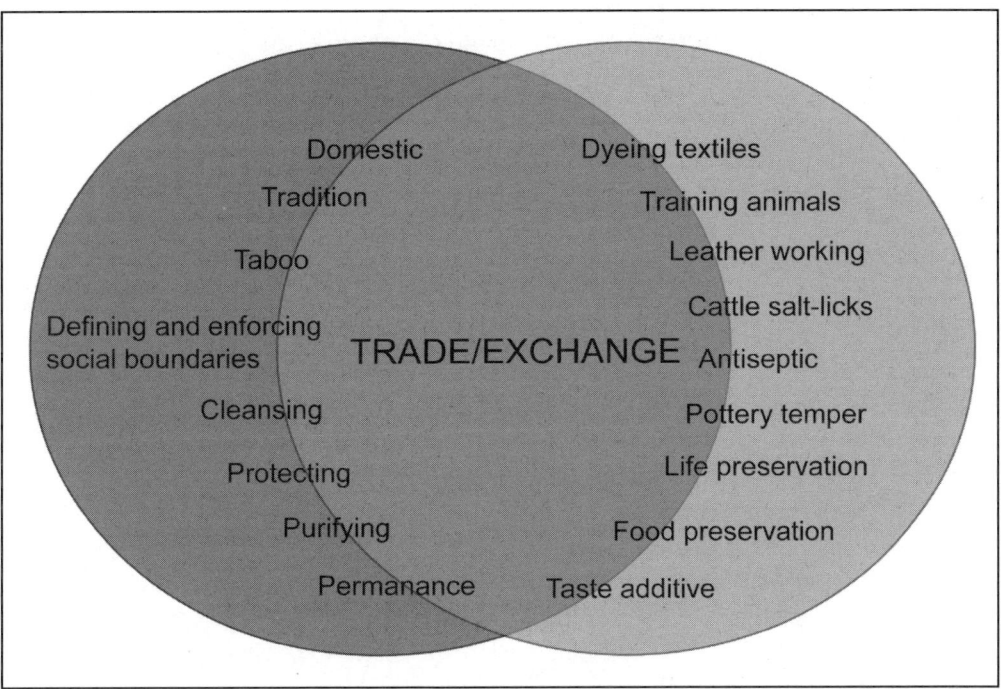

Figure 5.3. Uses of salt, derived from ethnographic and historical literature (left: traditional themes; right: practical uses).

of salt production. It is significant that, as yet, no evidence for the storage of whole containers for use in another season has been found on these sites.

To understand the very existence of salt production-sites, it is important to now explore salt consumption practices. Whilst the question of producers and consumers will not be explored in any detail here, it is useful to think about why salt was being produced in greater quantity during the Later Iron Age and Roman period in Britain.

> As an object of archaeology, salt leaves evidence fairly abundant for its production, and scarce for its consumption.
>
> (Adshead 1992, 4)

It is often assumed that salt was primarily produced to fulfil the need to preserve food, thus allowing greater freedom of movement and food insurance. Without doubt, a large part of the consumption of salt was for the preservation of foodstuffs: there is growing archaeological evidence that pork was being processed on some Late Iron Age salt production-sites (Maltby 2006).

Aside from preservation, salt can transform foodstuffs in other senses; it can change the taste and even enhance and change the colour of some meats from grey to pink.

Direct consumption of salt also has an effect on the human body, in that it makes people thirsty. If heavily-salted food, for example meat, was consumed during a meal, or even a feast, it would have required a lot of water (or perhaps other beverages including alcohol) to counteract this reaction.

Taste is an important element when considering individual and group consumption behaviour. Sensory experience of salt consumption includes the taste, texture, colour and translucency of the crystals but ideas of 'good salt' are culturally determined. For examples, seawater contains compounds, such as potassium chloride and magnesium sulphates, that impart a bitter taste (bittern) to the salt if not removed during the process (Gilman *et al.* 1998, 3). It is often assumed that, in the past, bittern would have been removed during the production process to make the salt more palatable, as is the case in modern times. However Denton (1984) observed that some traditional African tribes actually *prefer* this bitter taste. This is a reminder that we cannot simply project Western concepts of taste back onto past societies.

With diet and taste considered, how else could salt have been used and perceived in the past? Looking at ethnographic and historical research, it is clear that salt has had an even larger role to play, incorporating a variety of associated meanings and symbolism. As part of this research, key themes have been continuously observed in ethnographic and historical literature; these are represented on the left in figure 5.3. The possible 'practical uses' are represented on the right hand side.

The Meaning of Salt

Roud (2006, 387–393) details superstitions in Britain and Ireland associated with salt consumption. Although he considered evidence dating to the medieval and post-medieval period, it is notable how the main themes he raised are echoed across the world by different cultures: could they share common roots much earlier in human history? Spilling salt is probably the most famous superstition associated with salt, and is still adhered to by some. Roud (2006, 392) points out that in the earliest form of this superstition (at least 400 years ago), it was not the spiller of the salt that was unlucky; it was the person towards whom the salt fell. Salt superstitions are well preserved in regional folklore; for example a Somerset folklore describes how spreading salt on a front door-step will deter evil people from the house and prevent them from calling upon the inhabitants (Palmer 1976).

In this context it is useful to refer back to the case for the deposition of briquetage in pits in the north-east of England. A common theme for the symbolic use of salt throughout the historical record is to cleanse and protect from harm, as was emphasized by the case of the Somerset folklore. Could the deposition of this material, so closely associated with salt, have been symbolic of this house-cleansing and protecting ritual? Of course, in this case, only briquetage remains and it will never be clear if salt was also present. Perhaps because salt was a valuable commodity at this time, a material representative of salt was used instead. However, significantly, both acts of deposition were carried out at the end of the occupation of these structures, raising questions about this particular interpretation. Salt rarely appears to have represented the 'end', just the transformation into something else. Perhaps in this case it could have represented the transformation of the house into something else, the living to the dead, but not necessarily the end.

According to Roud (2006, 338) we should not to apply too much significance to the use of salt throughout history. This is because salt had many 'practical' uses that he considers to have been separate from any deeper 'hidden meanings'. In this sense, Roud sees a clear difference between the practical use of salt and the meanings that could become manifested in ritual or superstitious behaviour. Nenquin in his work on prehistoric salt production views the two as automatically intertwined:

> The salt which preserves the food, automatically becomes a symbol of eternity, constancy and force.
>
> (Nenquin 1961, 10).

Perhaps the two practices were mixed together, or treated separately, as appropriate to the meaning at the time. Attempting to elucidate different cultural attitudes and practice can be difficult because even if salt was involved in superstition or taboo, their meanings probably varied greatly across different cultures, communities and regions. Information that we have about modern and historic tradition, customs and superstition cannot be directly applied to the past but they do provide a tool to open up the discussion about the consumption of salt in past societies.

The cultural significance of water and of resources taken from the water is an important consideration when attempting to understand any potential meanings associated with salt consumption. Throughout European prehistory certain artefacts, particularly broken objects, were deliberately placed in springs, lakes and rivers (Bradley 1998; 2000). The act of depositing artefacts in water would appear to suggest that *giving* to watery places was significant. As with salt, water is essential to life and also provides a contrast with the dry, providing the arena for a variety of associations, meanings and contrasts (Bovin and Owac 2004). Sources of water can provide a natural focus for a community with a wide variety of potential meanings and significance. The idea of giving objects to the water is interesting in the light of salt production, an act that involves *taking* from a water source.

Freshwater could be consumed for water and seawater consumed for salt, both could be exploited for fish. It is often assumed that the sea in particular has always been a 'marine resource', much as we see it today, that can be freely exploited as needed for its contents. However this may not have always been the case. For instance, in Iron Age Britain, at a time when the extraction of salt from the sea increased, the consumption of fish appears to have been relatively low (Dobney and Eryynck 2007). This seems unusual as many coastal areas, such as Poole Harbour in Dorset, were teeming with production and trade activity during the Late Iron Age. Dobney and Eryynck (2007) argue that the dearth of fish bones on Iron Age sites cannot be explained by taphonomic factors and most probably reflects a deliberate avoidance of fish consumption. On mainland Europe, however, many Iron Age/Roman salt production-sites have been interpreted as 'pickling sites' for meat *and* fish (Nenquin 1961). If fish consumption was relatively 'off the menu' in Iron Age Britain, was this a matter of taste, or perhaps a taboo towards consuming living food from the sea? If water sources were perceived as special, symbolic or sacred in some way, did the act of consuming crystals taken from the sea become significant through association? Could this symbolism and meaning have been absorbed into the individual consuming salt?

Referring back to Roud's (2006, 338) suggestion that the 'practical' should be separated from deeper meanings, it seems possible that salt could have transcended a community's belief system, being viewed simply as a practical necessity. Essentially it depends on how integral any chosen symbolic associations were to a community as a whole and whether they could be used as and when needed, without being universally tied. However, it does appear that much of the behaviour during this period was greatly embedded in this belief system, and that this was integral to all aspects of everyday life.

Themes of permanence and preservation appear to have been incorporated into many belief systems throughout time and space (Fig. 5.3). With this in mind it is interesting to consider the partially-complete Roman lead salt-boiling container discovered on land in Shavington, South Cheshire (Penney and Shotter 1996). The container had been inscribed with the word 'VIVENTIUS', derived from the Latin word 'VIVIERE' meaning 'to live' or 'have life'. This symbolic association between salt and life is again seen in Balkan ethnography:

> Among the Saracatsans…in the case of the death of a new-born or a miscarriage there was a widespread custom…to put the child in a bag of salt and to hang it above the parents' marital bed for approximately forty days, until the child's corpse dries out. After this period the corpse of the deceased child… is buried in a pit dug in a corner of the hut…
>
> (Borić and Stefanović, 2004, 541)

Here salt represents preservation and permanence of life, even after death, perhaps helping to acknowledge and signify the transformation from life to death of the child. In this sense, this is the same theme that could have been symbolized by briquetage deposition observed at the Romano-British hut in Melsonby.

Conclusion
This paper has aimed to highlight just a few thoughts on the cultural significance of consuming salt in the past. The title of this paper 'Take it with a pinch of salt?' symbolizes two meanings. The first is to act as a reminder that choosing to incorporate

salt into our diet spans thousands of years. The second is intended to address the nature of inferring past cultural practices and behaviour through the exploration of examples in historical literature and ethnographic work. Although this research is primarily concerned with assessing the archaeological remains for salt production, it would only tell part of the story if the narrative was left there.

The holistic method of approaching this evidence, provides a view of the entire lifecycle of salt within prehistory and beyond, addressing not only the evidence for the actual sites and material used to produce salt, but also the ways that salt could be consumed, directly or indirectly. This approach therefore not only incorporates the physical archaeological evidence itself, but also considers the cultural behaviour which enabled this process to take place. Why people started producing salt and how it was subsequently consumed have been considered here to not only understand the technological choices employed for producing salt, but to also consider the cultural significance of the process. Adding inferences about aspects of past individual and cultural behaviour can only be a positive addition to the overall story of early salt production in Britain.

References

Adshead, S. A. M. 1992. *Salt and Civilisation* (London).
Borić, D. and Stefanović, S. 2004. 'Birth and death: infant burials from Vlasac and Lepenski Vir', *Antiquity* **78**, 526–546.
Bovin, N. and Owac, M. A. 2004. *Soils, Stones and Symbols: Cultural Perceptions of the Mineral World* (London).
Bradley, R. 1998. *The Passage of Arms: An Archaeological Analysis of Prehistoric Hoard and Votive Deposits* (Oxford).
Bradley, R. 2000. *An Archaeology of Natural Places* (London).
Chapman, J., Monah, D., Dumitroaia, G., Armstrong, H., Millard, A. and Francis, M. 2001. 'The exploitation of salt in the pre-history of Moldavia, Romania', *Archaeological Reports, University of Durham, for 1999/2000*, 10–20.
Chowne, P. 2001. *Excavations at Billingborough, Lincolnshire, 1975–8: A Bronze Age-Iron Age Settlement and Salt-working Site* (Salisbury).
De Brisay, K. W. 1975. 'The Red Hills of Essex', in De Brisay, K. W. and Evans, K. A. (eds.) *Salt: The Study of an Ancient Industry: Report on the Salt Weekend held at the University of Essex, 20–22 September 1974* (Colchester), 5–11
De Brisay, K. W. 1978. 'The excavation of a Red Hill at Peldon, Essex, with notes on other sites', *Antiquaries Journal* **58**, 31–60.
Denton, D. 1984. *The Hunger for Salt: An Anthropological, Physiological and Medical Analysis.* (New York).
Dobney, K. and Eryynck, A. 2007. 'To fish or not to fish? Evidence for the possible avoidance of fish consumption during the Iron Age around the North Sea', in Haselgrove, C. and Moore, T. (eds) *The Later Iron Age in Britain and Beyond* (Oxford), 403–418.
Fawn, A. J., Evans, K. A., McMaster, I. and Davis, G. M. R. 1990. *The Red Hills of Essex: Salt-Making in Antiquity* (Colchester).
Gilman, P., Barford, P., Fielding, A. and Penney, S. 1998. *Monuments Protection Programme. The Salt Industry*. Unpublished Step 1 Report for English Heritage. Consultation Report for April 1998, Essex County Council.

Grove, J. and Brunning, R. 1998. 'The Romano-British salt industry in Somerset', *Archaeology in The Severn Estuary* **9**, 61–68.

Lane, T. and Morris, E. L. 2001. *A Millennium of Saltmaking: Prehistoric and Romano-British Salt Production in the Fenland* (Sleaford).

Leech, R. H. 1981. 'The Somerset Levels in the Romano-British period', in Rowley, R. T. (ed.) *The Evolution of Marshland Lansdscapes. Papers Presented to a Conference on Marshland Landscapes December 1979* (Oxford), 20–51.

Maltby, M. 2006. 'Salt and animal products: linking production and use in Iron Age Britain', in Maltby, M. (ed.) *Integrating Zooarchaeology. Proceedings of the 9th Conference of the International Council of Archaeozoology* (Oxford).

Morris, E. L. 1994. 'Production and distribution of pottery and salt in Iron Age Britain: a review', *Proceedings of the Prehistoric Society* **60**, 371–393.

Nenquin, J. A. E. 1961. *Salt, a Study in Economic Prehistory: Dissertationes Archaeologicae Gandenses VI.* (Brugge).

Palmer, K. 1976. *The Folklore of Somerset* (London).

Penney, S. and Shotter, D. C. A. 1996. 'An inscribed Roman salt-pan from Shavington, Cheshire', *Britannia* **27**, 360–365.

Rippon, S. 2000. 'Exploitation and modification: changing patterns in the use of coastal resources in southern Britain during the Roman and medieval periods', in Aberg, A. and Lewis, C. (eds) *The Rising Tide: Archaeology and Coastal Landscapes* (Oxford), 65–75.

Roud, S., 2006. *The Penguin Guide to the Superstitions of Britain and Ireland* (London).

Sunter, N. and Woodward, P. J. 1987. *Romano-British Industries in Purbeck: Excavations at Norden. Excavations at Ower and Rope Lake Hole* (Dorchester).

Willis, S. 1999. 'Without and within: aspects of culture and community in the Iron Age of north-eastern England', in Bevan, B. (ed.) *Northern Exposure: Interpretative Devolution and the Iron Ages in Britain* (Leicester), 81–110.

The Distribution of the Catering Trade in Ostia Antica

Anna Kieburg,
Archäologisches Institut, University of Hamburg

Introduction
When Russell Meiggs (1960, 428) wrote his book about Roman Ostia he concluded his chapter on recreation by stating, 'in modern societies the inn, the bar, and the café are the main rivals of organized entertainment in the pattern of social recreation. The *caupona* and the *popina* took their place in Roman life.' This quotation makes plain one of the major problems of previous research concerning ancient gastronomy: the assumption that Roman professional catering can be directly compared with modern bars and restaurants. Recent research has demonstrated repeatedly the problems with drawing such analogies (e.g. MacMahon 2005; Ellis 2005) and there is a need to consider the evidence for the Roman catering trade on its own merits.

Traditionally, scholars have focused on the Pompeian or Campanian material and the evidence for the catering trade in Ostia Antica has been used only as comparison, if at all. Up to now, only Gustav Hermansen (1982, 126–83) has synthesized and analysed the Ostian data in detail but, because 25 years of research have been undertaken since the publication of his work, Hermansen's database now seems incomplete and the catering trade of Roman Ostia requires a new examination (Kieburg forthcoming). By examining the taverns and lodgings in Roman towns, this paper aims to illustrate the exceptional situation in the ancient city of Ostia Antica with the goal of interpreting the function of urban catering and its role in wider Roman economy and society. Here the term tavern will be used to refer to catering outlets and specific references to properties in Ostia follow Hermansen's (1982) numbering system (1–38) by which all 38 of Ostia's taverns have been catalogued.

Remains of the Catering Trade in Ostia
Excavations at Ostia in the early twentieth century brought to light examples of masonry structures that excavators compared immediately with similar structures from the sites of Pompeii and Herculaneum (*Notizie degli Scavi di Antichità*, Rome [hereafter *NSc*] 1915, 27–31) and identified as counters for outlets selling food and drink. Most were typical retail outlets with wide openings to a street or portico for commercial activities while the rear of a unit may have been used for serving, storage and/or accommodation. Of the 38 identified catering units, there are six – no. 5: Reg. I 10,2; no. 9: Reg. II 2,2 east; no. 25: Reg. III 17,5; nos. 30 and 31: Reg. IV 5,7; and no. 37: Reg. V 4,1 (see Hermansen 1982, 134–78) – of which nothing can be seen today but

The Distribution of the Catering Trade in Ostia Antica

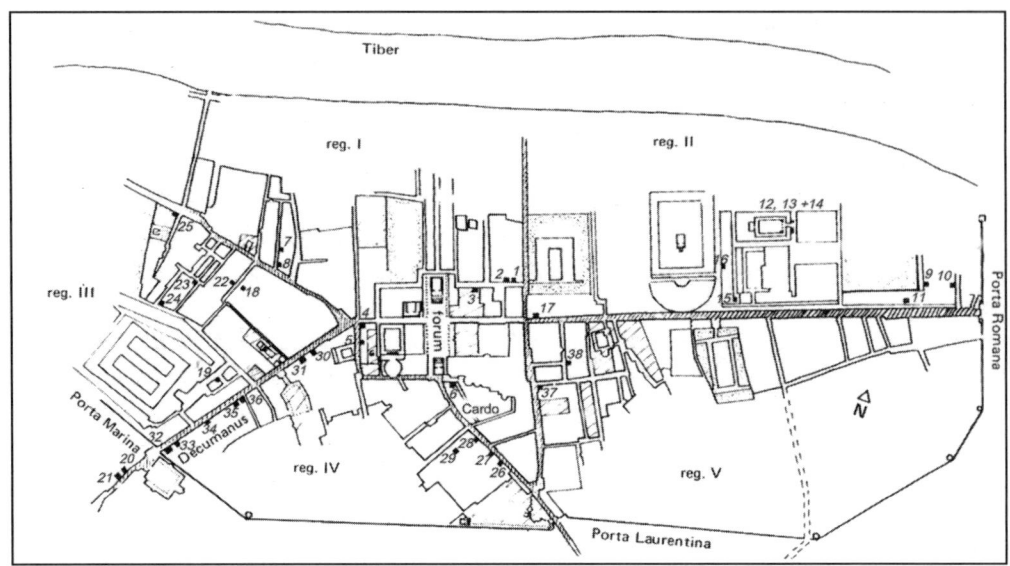

Figure 6.1. Map of Ancient Ostia (scale 1:7500). The location of taverns are marked in black squares numbering 1–38 (after Hermansen 1982: fig. 2).

they are classified as taverns because counter structures are recorded in the original plans of Italo Gismondi (Calza 1953, plans 1–14).

Mosaics have been used to identify a further four catering units and these are still visible today. Three are adjacent to the casern of the *vigils* (nos. 12–14: Reg. II 5,1) and the fourth, found at property no. 15: Reg. II 6,1, is located directly on the intersection of the Decumanus and the Via della Fontana (see *NSc* 1909: 92; Becatti 1953, 62–63, Tav. CXCII, 78–80; Hermansen 1982: 143–47). The last mosaic bears the message *[HOSPES INQUIT] FORTUNATUS [VINVM ET CR]ATERA QUOD SITIS BIBE*, inviting passers-by to stop and have a drink (Zangenmeister 1871 XIV, S 4756). This, together with representations of vases/drinking vessels on the mosaics in nos. 13 and 14, strongly indicate that these properties represent taverns. It is curious, however, that there are no instances where significant mosaics and counter structures exist together.

The remaining 27 catering outlets are identified by counter structures. Approximately half of these are in a very poor condition; in most cases only the shelf elements or basins from the brick-built counter have survived and only a few have been preserved or reconstructed. The counters are commonly covered with marble fragments (e.g. no. 3: Reg. I 2,3–5; no. 19: Reg. III 5,1 and no. 26: Reg. IV 2,3) or coloured stucco, as at no. 29: Reg. IV 2,6, the so-called *Caupona del Pavone*.

Examining the distribution of taverns may help to elucidate why there are so few catering outlets compared to Campanian towns. On first view, the plan of Ostia (Fig. 6.1) shows a rather scattered distribution of taverns. This contrasts with the high density of catering outlets at Pompeii where, according to Laurence (1994, 70–84),

The Distribution of the Catering Trade in Ostia Antica

these encouraged the streets to be full of deviant behaviour: drinking, gambling and prostitution. However, remains of the catering trade are actually found in every important place at Ostia: at the commercial centres of the *horrea* (Region II 2,2 east and west), near temples (e.g. Region III 17,5), on the main streets (e.g. Regions II 2,6 and II 9,2), close to rich houses (e.g. Regions III 5,1 and III 14,1), next to public baths (Regions I 12,10 and III 10,2), the theatre (Region II 6,5), the forum (Region I 10,2) and the city gates (Regions III 7,3 and IV 7,4). Faced with the density of retail units (more than 800 in the excavated areas of Ostia), the total of only 38 catering trade outlets seems small, considering that much of Ostia's population, permanent and temporary alike, relied heavily on food and drink obtained from outlets to fulfil their needs (DeLaine 2005, 30). Even after the extensive rebuilding phase during the reign of Domitian, including the construction of more domestic cooking and sanitary facilities, taverns must have remained a common feature of Ostian streets (Meiggs 1960, 64–78).

To obtain a clear understanding of Ostia's catering trade and the role it played in commercial and daily life requires that the spatial pattern of the taverns is examined in detail; the sections below attempt to do precisely this.

Tavern Distribution in Minor Areas

Many of Ostia's catering outlets were located in minor or dead-end streets, not visible from the major thoroughfares, as for example the taverns no. 18: Reg. III 1,10 near the Bath of the Seven Sages; no. 23: Reg. III 1,10 in the Via degli Tecti Aurighi; and nos 12–14: Reg. II 5,1 at the caserns of the *vigils* (see Becatti 1953, 125–6; Hermansen 1982, 143–51). To find them would, therefore, have required a degree of local knowledge. It is possible that these taverns operated as catering-services for nearby public or semi-private areas like baths, *collegia* and the caserns of the *vigils*. If this were the case, they would have required large areas for the preparation and storage of food. Until such aspects are examined by scholars, definitive statements on this point cannot be made.

Tavern Distribution in Major Public Areas

Located in close proximity to the forum were just four taverns: no. 3: Region I 2,3–5; no. 4: Region I 10,1; no. 5: Region I 10,2; no. 6: Region I 12,10 (see *NSc* 1916: 143, 399–428; Kleberg 1957, 46; Calza and Nash 1959, 79; Hermansen 1982, 130–135). Only nos. 3 and 6 have direct access to the forum, a much lower figure than the catering outlets around the forum at Pompeii, where five taverns are found at the north, and three at the south end of the forum (Fig. 6.1 and see Ellis 2004, 376–7, Fig. 3; 2005, 124).

The biggest street intersection in Ostia, of the Decumanus and the Via della Foce, has only two immediately accessible taverns; again, unlike the big intersections in Pompeii (Ellis 2004, 379–80; Ellis 2005, 133–8). Similarly, taverns are absent around Ostia's theatre, the Piazza dei Corporazioni and, most significantly, along the whole eastern Decumanus from the Porta Romana to the forum.

The Distribution of the Catering Trade in Ostia Antica

This apparent lack of evidence for the catering trade in major public areas may not reflect reality; instead it may be a result of the slow decline of the ancient city combined with the hurried excavations of Guido Calza and Giovanni Becatti in the 1930s. It is possible to imagine, for instance, that as the city began to wane during the fourth century, the catering units gradually fell out of use and decayed, their building materials being re-used and their structures becoming eroded by natural processes. By the time they came to be excavated, much of the evidence necessary for their classification as 'tavern' would already have been lost. After excavation, poor conservation has accelerated the loss of information about the catering trade: even in the last 50 years several of the taverns identified in Gismondi's plans have become unrecognizable (Calza 1953). It may, therefore, be assumed that many more of Ostia's retail outlets were connected to the catering trade than has been recognized to date; the situation may actually have been closer to that seen at Pompeii.

Pompeii, in particular the areas around the city gates, provides a good case-study for understanding the importance of taverns within the urban economy. The evidence from this city also has the potential to help interpret the catering-trade remains in Ostia. As Steven Ellis (2004, 381) has demonstrated, along Pompeii's Via Stabiana, near to the Porta di Stabia gate, there were as many as 13 retail counters, all along the east side of the street (one approximately every 17 metres). Twelve of these 13 counters were located on the north side of each property's threshold, clearly visible to pedestrians on their way to the town centre. The tendency to align counters with areas of greatest activity and movement probably indicates the directional flow of ambulatory traffic, about which we might otherwise have little knowledge. This information shows that the spatial arrangement of Pompeii was partly guided by forces of economic rationality, as Ellis (2004, 383) concludes:

> Bars were fundamental features of the Roman daily life, and eager protagonists in the ancient economy, as is demonstrated by their distribution in areas of greatest social activity. We can recognize how, in the spatial arrangement and alignment of their facades and counters, bars competed between themselves for the custom of people entering the town and of those who gathered about a street corner. Bars and their counters were not randomly configured. Their arrangements can help to illustrate systems of urban behaviour.

So, it would advance the research of the Ostian catering trade considerably if this 'Pompeian pattern' of profit-oriented counter positioning could be identified at Ostia. Whilst the archaeological evidence at Ostia is not as well preserved as at Pompeii, the two cities demonstrate similarities in terms of their retail unit architecture and placement. As such it should be possible to compare the Ostian with the Pompeian remains.

The Distribution of the Catering Trade in Ostia Antica

The Distribution along Main Streets

In Ostia, just two areas have provided sufficient evidence of catering outlets to allow the 'Pompeian pattern' to be considered: the first is the southern *cardo maximus*, leading from the Porta Laurentina to the forum, and the second is the western part of the Decumanus, leading from the Porta Marina to the intersection with the Via della Foce (for a ground-plan of the whole western Decumanus see Gismondi's plans in Calza 1953).

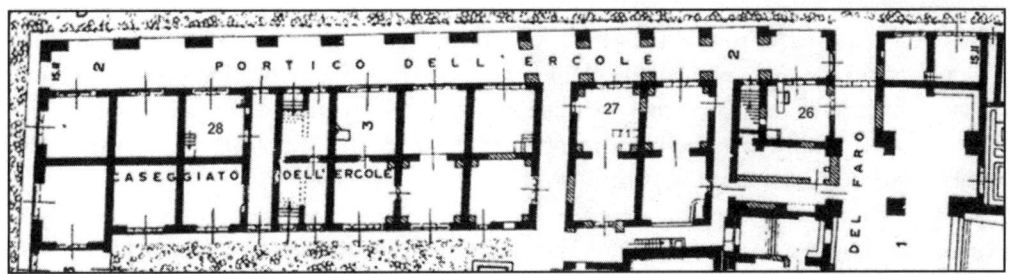

Figure 6.2. Ground plan of the Porticus of Hercules with taverns nos. 26, 27 and 28 (after Gismondi in Calza 1953).

Three taverns are located along the southern *cardo maximus* (Fig. 6.2). Tavern no. 26: Reg. IV 2,3, can be seen from the city gate and is well positioned near the entrance to the Bath of Pharus (see Hermansen 1982, 16). The counter has the characteristic L-form, is covered with decorative marble plates and has the typical Ostian mid-set basin. The counter is oriented to attract passing traffic entering the town; however, a second entrance to this tavern from the *fauces* of the aforementioned bath would have increased the flow of customers. Further north is the second tavern, no. 27: Region IV 2,3 (Hermansen 1982, 163–4) located in the Porticus of Hercules. Here the counter is similar in form to that at tavern no. 26 but its positioning within the property is different; it lies at the rear of the room and is not visible from the exterior. It does not invite passers-by to drink or snack, but presumes a local knowledge and, thus, is not directed at traffic entering the town.

The third tavern, no. 28: Region IV 2,3 (Hermansen 1982, 165–7) also within the Porticus of Hercules, requires closer evaluation. The remains show little comparable to a counter, only the stepped shelves that are known from other Ostian and Pompeian taverns (Fig. 6.3). The question which arises from this particular property is the same for other taverns in Ostia: how could food and drink be served here with so little workspace? One possibility is that a counter extension was constructed in front of the shelves and towards the entrance of the tavern; a hypothetical reconstruction of this is shown in figure 6.4. This would not have been in full sight of customers coming up the street from the Porta Laurentina but would have attracted traffic coming from the direction of the forum. Although no remains have been found to indicate that such an

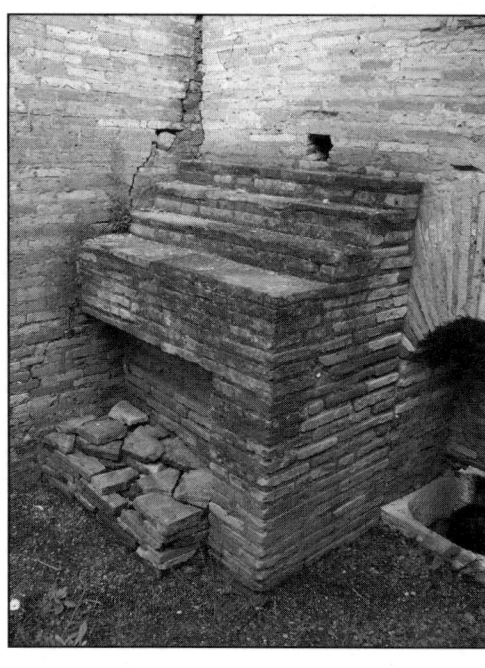

Figure 6.3. Rebuilt shelf element in tavern no. 28. Photograph by A. Kieburg.

extension existed at this property, similar counters have been found in taverns no. 3: Region I 2,3–5 (see *NSc* 1916, 143, 399–428; Kleberg 1957, 46; Calza and Nash 1959, 79) and no. 29.

In all, the three taverns nos. 26, 27 and 28 show differing orientation of counters and only one, no. 26, lies in full sight of traffic entering the city. Although there are many retail units along both sides of the *cardo maximus*, it remains to be hypothesized whether or not there were more catering taverns in this area. The differing position of the remaining counters does not let us transfer the 'Pompeian pattern' of profit-orientation to this part of Ostia. The direction of ambulatory traffic remains shrouded and it is not possible to reconstruct the catering-trade economy in the area around the Porta Laurentina.

The sample size for the second area, the western part of the Decumanus, is larger, with seven examples of taverns (nos. 30–36), but the remains are in a poor state of conservation. Interestingly, all seven taverns are situated to the right-hand side of traffic entering the town from the shore and no catering outlets have been identified on the opposite side of the street, the same phenomenon seen along the Via Stabiana in Pompeii. In both no. 30: Region IV 5,7 east and no. 31: Region IV 5,7 west (Hermansen 1982, 169–72) no remnants of the counter structures shown in Gismondi's plans have survived (see Calza 1953). In no. 32: Region IV 7,4 (Hermansen 1982, 172–5), the so-called Caupona di Alexander Helix, the built-in stepped shelves and basins remain visible today. At no. 33: Region IV 7,3 and nos. 34–36: Region IV 7,2 (Hermansen

The Distribution of the Catering Trade in Ostia Antica

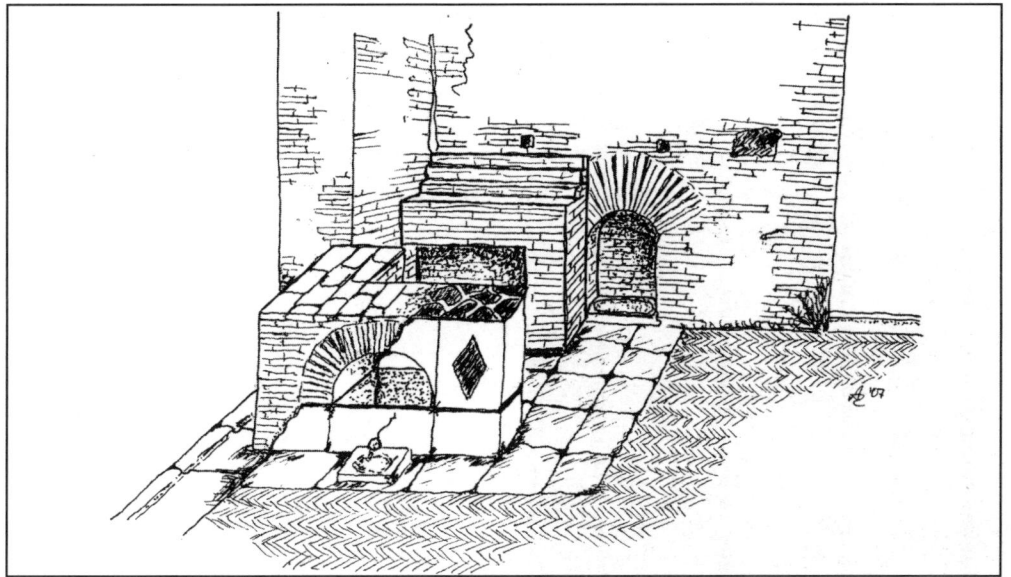

Figure 6.4. Hypothetical reconstruction of an additional counter element in tavern no. 28. Drawing by A. Kieburg.

1982, 175–77) only fragments of basin elements remain. The actual appearance of the counters and their orientation is only hypothetical in some cases, but the available evidence points to an orientation allowing full side-views from the entrance. With the exception of no. 34, counters were sited purposely according to the direction of potential customers coming from the Porta Marina to the city centre, demonstrating economic efficiency and ambulatory flow. In this case the density of taverns and the position of the counter remains does seem to suggest the profit-oriented 'Pompeian pattern'.

Conclusion

The remains of the Ostian catering trade can provide only a restricted view of daily tavern life and its economic importance in the city. Despite the high density of *retail units* along the streets and other areas, the archaeological evidence suggests no more than 38 taverns, a very low number for a city such as Ostia. It seems possible that many more of the 'retail outlets' in the highly-frequented areas of the forum, baths, theatre and section of main routes were actually taverns and that the density of these catering outlets was more akin to that seen in Pompeii.

Having examined two areas where a sufficient density of catering-trade outlets survives, only along the western Decumanus can the spatial arrangement of taverns be demonstrated to reflect the profit-oriented 'Pompeian pattern'. The evidence indicates competition between the taverns for the custom of people entering the town and illustrates the direction of ambulatory flow from the harbour to the city centre. A lack of evidence of private cooking facilities points to the high importance for food and drink outlets not only for many permanent residents but also for travellers, merchants, craftsmen and day-labourers. So, despite the archaeologically-restricted view of tavern life in Ostia Antica, it is evident that taverns were exceedingly important for basic daily provisions, and so were a cornerstone of the urban economy rather than being places for mere entertainment and recreation.

References

Becatti, G. 1953. *Scavi di Ostia IV: Mosaici e Pavimenti Marmorei* (Rome).
Calza, G. 1953. *Scavi di Ostia I: Topografia Generale* (Rome).
Calza, R. and Nash, E. 1959. *Ostia* (Florence).
DeLaine, J. 2005. 'The commercial landscape of Ostia', in MacMahon, A. and Price, J. (eds) *Roman Working Lives and Urban Living* (Oxford) 29–47.
Ellis, S. J. R. 2004. 'The distribution of bars in Pompeii: archaeological, spatial and viewshed analyses', *Journal of Roman Archaeology* **17**, 371–84.
Ellis, S. J. R. 2005. *The Pompeian Bar and the City: Defining Food and Drink Outlets and Identifying their Place in the Urban Environment*. Unpublished PhD thesis, University of Sydney.
Hermansen, G. 1982. *Ostia: Aspects of Roman City Life* (Edmonton).
Kieburg, A. forthcoming. *Betrachtungen zum Römischen Gastronomiegewerbe in Pompeji, Herkulaneum und Ostia*. Unpublished PhD thesis, University of Hamburg.
Kleberg, T. 1957. *Hôtels, Restaurants et Cabarets dans l'Antiquité Romain* (Uppsala).
Laurence, R. 1994. *Roman Pompeii: Space and Society* (London).
MacMahon, A. 2005. 'The *taberna* counters of Pompeii and Herculaneum', in MacMahon, A. and Price, J. (eds) *Roman Working Lives and Urban Living* (Oxford), 70–87.
Meiggs, R. 1960. *Roman Ostia* (Oxford).
Pavolini, C. 1991. *La Vita Quotidiana a Ostia* (Rome-Bari).
Wallace-Hadrill, A. 1994. *Houses and Society in Pompeii and Herculaneum* (Princeton).
Zangenmeister, C. 1871. *Corpus Inscriptionum Latinarum IV* (Berlin).

Medieval Diet: Evidence for a London Signature?

Kay Lakin,
University of Reading

Introduction

This paper considers the period from the Norman invasion (1066) until the Reformation, *ca.* 1540. During this time, the types of food consumed were influenced by a variety of factors – socio-economics, religion and geography – and different populations consumed different types of food (see Woolgar *et al.* 2006). Medieval documents detail the foodstuffs grown, bought and served in larger households which, along with archaeological studies of animal and plant remains, have provided a good picture of medieval diet. These traditional methods of analysis, however, provide only a general indication of broad changes in medieval diet and there is still a great deal that is not known about how individual and group diets changed through time. Chemical analysis of human remains has the potential to provide new information about long-term diet at the level of the individual, to identify, for example, individuals from the same site who due to wealth or status had different diets from the rest of the population under study.

Up to now stable isotope analysis has provided evidence to suggest that late-medieval individuals had a different dietary signature than those from earlier historic and Prehistoric periods. This dietary change has further implications because it suggests an alteration in attitude towards certain types of food. To date, however, all interpretations of diet using stable isotope analyses are from sites in the north of England (Fuller *et al.* 2006; Fuller *et al.* 2003; Mays 1997; Mays *et al.* 2002; Müldner and Richards 2005; Müldner and Richards 2007a; Richards *et al.* 2002). Therefore, we might expect to see a different isotopic pattern emerge for the south, especially London.

This study will test whether diet in later medieval London was isotopically different to that from earlier periods or that suggested by analyses for the north of England. To achieve this, 150 individuals from the site of the former hospital and priory of St Mary without Bishopsgate (St Mary Spital) have been analysed in order to see if a London-based diet can be identified within the sampled population. Over 10,000 individuals have been uncovered during the excavations of the hospital, making it the largest collection ever recovered from a single site. A substantial number have been osteologically assessed, making this collection an invaluable resource in order to explore medieval diet. Moreover, these individuals come from a single period of the hospital, when it was prosperous and a great number of people from different backgrounds may have been buried there.

Principles of Stable Isotopes for Diet Reconstruction

The use of stable isotopes to reconstruct past diet relies on the principle that we are what we eat. Protein, fat and carbohydrate in food are incorporated into our bodily tissues, including bone, which contain isotopes of carbon and nitrogen of specific ratios. Isotopes are atoms of an element with a different atomic number; that is, they differ by the number of neutrons in the nucleus and therefore, to a small degree, in their atomic weight. Due to a difference in the abundance of each isotope in nature, an isotope of low abundance (e.g. ^{13}C) is compared to the isotope of high abundance (e.g. ^{12}C) as a ratio ($^{13}C/^{12}C$ and $^{15}N/^{14}N$). It is these two ratios that are measured within skeletal tissues, most often in bone collagen, in order to reconstruct an individual's diet.

The food we eat contains a carbon and nitrogen isotopic signature, which has been passed through the food chain. Terrestrial and aquatic ecosystems have different isotopic signatures providing the possibility of identifying the type of food that has been consumed (see Fig. 7.1). The carbon dietary signature in a temperate climate, where plants of the C_3 photosynthetic pathway prevail, is used to distinguish between marine and terrestrial sources of food (Chisholm *et al.* 1982). The nitrogen dietary signature may also be used to identify aquatic and terrestrial food sources (Schoeninger and DeNiro 1984), but it mainly distinguishes between plant and animal foods in the diet (Sealy 2001). The combination of both isotope systems provides the opportunity

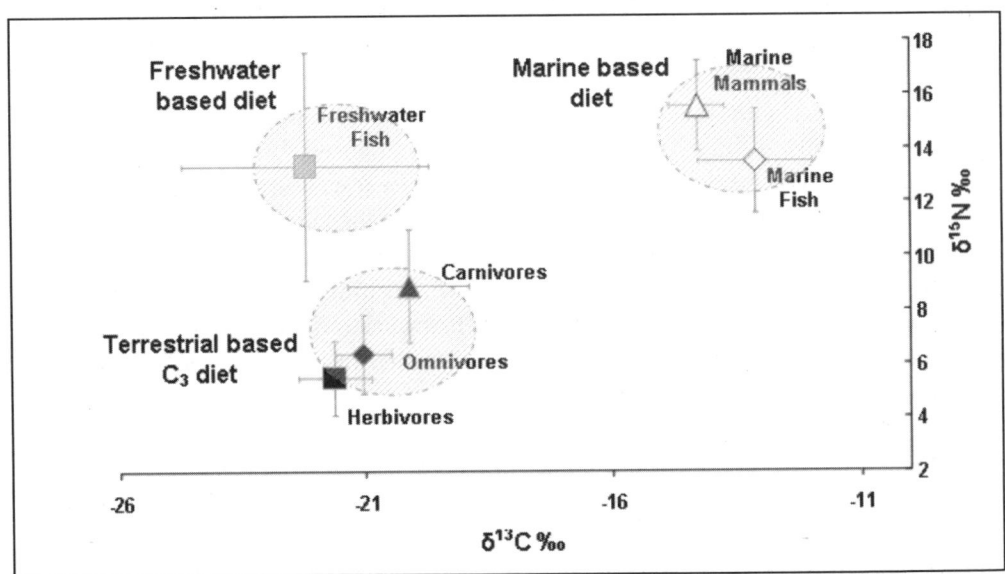

Figure 7.1. Isotopic map. The horizontal axis shows the carbon isotope dietary signature ($\delta^{13}C$ ‰), and the vertical axis the nitrogen isotope dietary signature ($\delta^{15}N$ ‰). Faunal isotope data were plotted from Müldner and Richards (2005) and Coltrain et al. (2004).

to identify freshwater food sources whose signatures are influenced by terrestrial carbon but whose nitrogen isotope ratios are closer to those of marine organisms (Beaudoin *et al.* 1999; Müldner and Richards 2005).

As with every technique for reconstructing diet in the past, there are some important methodological limitations. First, because bone collagen is analysed, the dietary signal reflects mainly the protein portion of the diet and not diet as a whole (Ambrose and Norr 1993). Second, due to the formation and subsequent slow turnover of bone, the isotope signature represents an average of the food consumed over the last 10–30 years before the death of the individual (Hedges *et al.* 2007). Lastly, the technique cannot be used to distinguish between different sources of protein that have the same position in the food web or between different by-products of the same animal; for instance between sheep and cattle, or between meat and milk (O'Connell and Hedges 1999). Despite these limitations, the technique is well established and has been used repeatedly to reconstruct successfully the past diet of individuals and populations from different periods and geographical areas. It is, however, most useful if it is used in conjunction with other methods of dietary reconstruction.

Medieval Diet: The Documentary and Archaeological Evidence

Commercialization developed rapidly through the course of the medieval period, directly impacting on diet. Cattle and sheep were increasingly raised for secondary products, including milk, while the burgeoning fishing industry provided inland communities with access to marine fish (Barrett *et al.* 2004). Although the major component of medieval diet was grain (usually in the form of bread or pottage) this was supplemented by meat and fish, the amounts consumed increasing with wealth and social position (Dyer 1989, 56). Christianity also influenced diet, dictating periods of abstinence, such as Lent, when the consumption of meat was forbidden but fish and/or dairy products could be consumed (see Harvey 1993, 61–2; Dawson this volume). Barrett *et al.* (2004) have suggested that the demand for fish during periods of fast may have instigated the international upsurge in marine fishing leading to a decline in the consumption of freshwater fish. While marine fish were generally more affordable and consumed more widely, freshwater fish were consumed by the most noble households and wealthy monastic inhabitants.

A number of catastrophic events, such as famines and plagues, notably the Black Death, had a significant effect on population sizes and therefore on standards of living. Documentary evidence suggests that the standards of living increased in the aftermath of the Black Death, most notably in the low-status communities where meat made a much larger contribution to the diet than before (Dyer 1989, 159).

In summary, different sectors of the medieval population consumed different quantities of plant, terrestrial and aquatic protein, with individuals of greater wealth consuming more animal protein, in the form of meat and fish, than the poor. This suggests that different social groups could potentially be identified based on the contribution of these different protein sources to the diet. Despite the varied and dynamic nature of medieval diet, very few British isotopic studies have centred on this period; the majority focusing on Prehistoric diets.

Medieval Isotopes: The Story So Far…
Simon Mays (1997) conducted one of the first published isotopic studies on English medieval diet. Using only the carbon isotope ratio, he suggested that individuals from different site-types in north-east England (Fishergate, York; Wharram Percy; Greyfriars, Hartlepool; Blackfriars, Newcastle; Castle Hill, Scarborough) consumed a terrestrial C_3 based diet with a small contribution of marine protein. He also observed differences between groups interred at the cemetery of Fishergate, York; the monastic community consuming greater proportions of marine food than the apparently wealthy lay individuals. Whilst Mays' results agree with the documentary evidence for high fish consumption by medieval religious communities, a recent re-analysis of the Fishergate population (Müldner and Richards 2007a) suggested that the observed differences were more probably linked to variations between the diets of males and females, males having consumed slightly more marine protein on average. Müldner and Richards' study was unable to detect differences between individuals of different social status, suggesting that the diets were not isotopically distinct. However, one group of individuals that exhibited perimortem blade injuries had unusual isotopic ratios, suggesting minimal marine protein in the diet, in contrast to the rest of the individuals analysed (Müldner and Richards 2007a). Such individuals may not have been identified based on their diet using traditional methods of dietary reconstruction.

Chemical analysis has also indicated that later medieval English diet was quite different to that from earlier periods, being characterized by slightly less negative carbon isotope values, but much higher nitrogen isotope values than earlier historic periods (Müldner and Richards 2005). The unusual stable isotope signal observed in later medieval populations still warrants further investigation, although Müldner and Richards (2007b) argue that the religious fasts, during which periods the consumption of meat was prohibited, increased the consumption of marine food in the diet. Furthermore, the fact that pigs were frequently fed animal products may have contributed to unusually high nitrogen values, while the availability of other ^{15}N enriched foods such as freshwater fish, poultry, eggs and molluscs may have also had an impact (Müldner and Richards 2007b). One later medieval site however, plots outside the usual range of later medieval isotope data: the rural village of Wharram Percy, York, whose cemetery population is thought to represent the local peasants. The inhabitants of this rural site appear to have consumed far less protein than the rest of the population and little marine fish. It seems therefore that stable isotope analysis is able to detect dietary differences between urban and rural communities, between low- and high-status sites but also individual variations in consumption. Traditional methods of dietary reconstruction could not provide this level of resolution and, with this in mind, it seems

Medieval Diet: Evidence for a London Signature?

possible that stable isotope analysis can provide important insights into the diets of a population that, on the surface, appears homogenous.

A London Diet? Evidence from the Hospital and Priory of St Mary Spital

Recently, London has become the subject of an important history-based study of diet: the 'Feeding a City' project which resulted in a number of publications based on documentary evidence (Galloway 1996; 1998; Galloway and Murphy 1991). As the metropolis, London had a very special status. Documentary sources indicate that London had a wide catchment radius with a high migrant population (Russell 1959; Thrupp 1989). This suggests that the city contained individuals from a variety of different social backgrounds and cultures, with equally diverse consumption practices. Diet in medieval London has not, however, been studied isotopically, a situation that this research seeks to redress.

St Mary without Bishopsgate, later known as St Mary Spital, became one of England's largest medieval hospitals, second only to St Leonard's in York. At its foundation, ca. 1197, it was a fairly humble hospital just to the north of Bishopsgate, probably consisting of the typical infirmary hall-style building often constructed at this time with possibly twelve or thirteen inmates (Thomas et al. 1997, 25). Throughout its life the hospital expanded and became more consistent with monastic institutions containing the typical cloistral ranges and the infirmary extended to two storeys. At the end of the fourteenth century, the economy of the hospital began to dwindle but it carried on until its dissolution in the early sixteenth century (Thomas et al. 1997, 78).

The hospital catered for both sexes and was known to take in pregnant women and provided care for their children if they died (Thomas et al. 1997, 39). It also provided hospitality to travellers to the city and beyond due to its north-bound suburban location (Orme and Webster 1995, 62). Whilst the hospital cemetery was used for the burial of inmates, lay brothers and sisters, canons, priests and masters, the large number of inhumations suggests that the hospital acted as an over-flow cemetery for the city as a whole, particularly during periods of epidemic (Thomas 2002, 48). As a priory it would have attracted wealthy individuals, and documentary evidence suggests that many wills requested a burial within the hospital grounds (Thomas et al. 1997, 123). Hospitals were also known to bury those who had not been baptized or were ostracized from the community (Orme and Webster 1995; Rawcliffe 1995). This evidence suggests that the cemetery of St Mary Spital was very mixed, containing individuals from a variety of backgrounds. If the hospital acted as an overflow cemetery for inner-city London, it may be assumed that many of the individuals buried there were inhabitants of London, which is important to the possible identification of a London-based diet.

Preliminary data from St Mary Spital suggest no such London diet, in fact the mean value plots within the range of the late-medieval sites from the north of England (Fig. 7.2). This suggests that the inhabitants of medieval London consumed a diet that was isotopically similar to other parts of England at this time. This does

Medieval Diet: Evidence for a London Signature?

not suggest, however, that there were no dietary differences between the north and south of England. Potentially, differences may have existed as to the types of meat or grain consumed, which cannot be resolved isotopically. Still, this result is interesting because it suggests an isotopically uniform diet, with the exception of Wharram Percy, throughout medieval England.

Conclusions and Future Research

It would seem that the average dietary isotopic signature of the sample of individuals analysed from St Mary Spital substantiate the work of Müldner and Richards (2005; 2007b), indicating a widespread dietary change into the late-medieval period. What is still unknown is when this change occurred and how prominent it was throughout society. In order to answer such questions, individuals buried from earlier phases of the hospital will be analysed for diachronic trends. In addition to work on this monastic institution, a second site – the parish church of St Nicholas Shambles – will also be analysed. The St Nicholas Shambles cemetery is not likely to be as mixed as that of St Mary Spital, but probably represents a distinct community within London – the traders

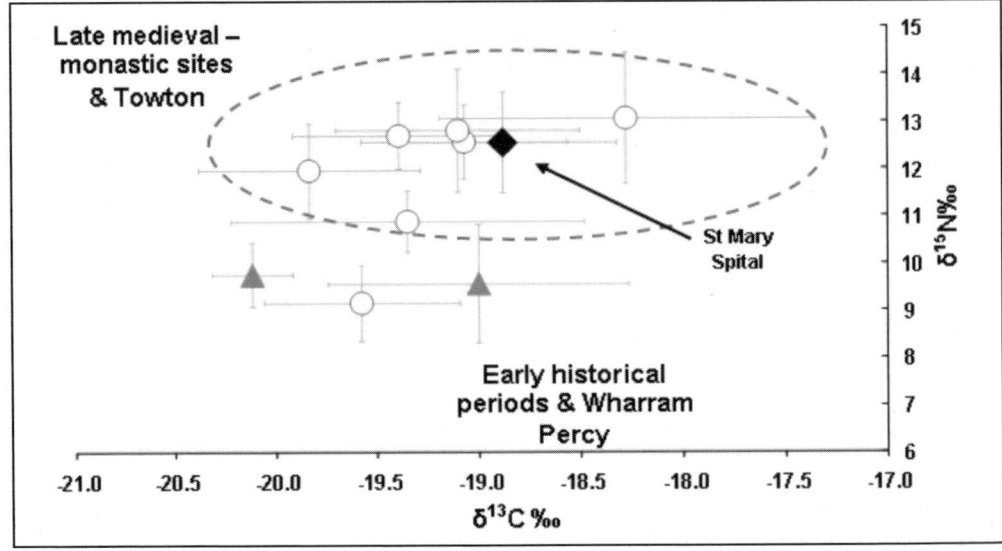

Figure 7.2. Human isotope data for six late-medieval sites, St Giles by Brompton Bridge, Warrington, Towton, St Andrews at Fishergate, Wharram Percy and Orkney (open circle symbols), and St Mary Spital (back diamond). The grey triangles are from two earlier periods, the Roman site of Poundbury camp, and the Anglo Saxon site Berinsfield. Notice the high nitrogen values of late-medieval sites, contained within the ellipse, and the low mean nitrogen value of Wharram Percy, which plots within the range of the earlier sites. Data plotted from Fuller et al. (2002), Müldner and Richards (2005; 2007a), Privat et al. (2002), Richards et al. (2006) and Richards et al. (1998).

(Schofield 1997). It is one of the few non-monastic cemeteries excavated within the London area and therefore provides a valuable comparison not only to St Mary Spital but also to other isotopic data-sets from medieval Britain, which are mostly derived from ecclesiastic sites. Moreover, the individuals buried in St Nicholas Shambles date slightly earlier than those from the hospital, providing the opportunity to examine whether AD 1000 was a watershed in diet, as suggested by Barrett *et al.* (2004) and observed in York (Müldner and Richards, 2007b). Moreover, sex, burial treatment and age will be compared within each site in order to address factors of social rank and identity.

References

Ambrose, S. H. and Norr, L. 1993. 'Experimental evidence for the relationship of the carbon isotope ratios of whole diet and dietary protein to those of bone collagen and carbonate', in Lambert, J. B. and Grupe, G. (ed.) *Prehistoric Human Bone: Archaeology at the Molecular Level* (Berlin), 1–37.

Barrett, J. H., Locker, A. M. and Roberts, C. M. 2004. ''Dark Age Economics' revisited: the English fish bone evidence AD 600–1600', *Antiquity* **78**, 618–636.

Beaudoin, C. P., Tonn, W. M., Prepas, E. E. and Wassenaar, L. I. 1999. 'Individual specialisation and trophic adaptability of northern pike (*Esox lucius*): an isotope and dietary analysis', *Oecologia* **120**, 386–396.

Chisholm, B. S., Nelson, D. E. and Schwarcz, H. P. 1982. 'Stable-carbon isotope ratios as a measure of marine versus terrestrial protein in ancient diets', *Science* **216**, 1131–1132.

Coltrain, J. B., Hayes, M. G. and O'Rourke, D. H. 2004. 'Sealing, whaling and caribou: the skeletal isotope chemistry of Eastern Arctic foragers', *Journal of Archaeological Science* **31**, 39–57.

Dyer, C. 1989: *Standards of Living in the Later Middle Ages: Social Change in England c. 1200–1520* (Cambridge).

Fuller, B. T., Richards, M. P. and Mays, S. A. 2003. 'Stable carbon and nitrogen variations in tooth dentine serial sections from Wharram Percy', *Journal of Archaeological Science* **30**, 1673–1684.

Fuller, B. T., Molleson, T. I., Harrison, L. T., Gilmour, L. T. and Hedges, R. E. M. 2006. 'Isotopic evidence for breastfeeding and possible adult dietary differences from Late/Sub-Roman Britain', *American Journal of Physical Anthropology* **129**, 45–54.

Galloway, J. 1996. 'London's grain supply: changes in production, distribution and consumption during the fourteenth century', *Franco-British Studies* **20**, 23–34.

Galloway, J.A. 1998. 'Driven by drink? Ale consumption and the agrarian economy of the London region ca. 1300–1400', in Carlin, M. and Rosenthal, J. T. (ed.) *Food and Eating in Medieval Europe* (London), 87–100.

Galloway, J. and Murphy, M. 1991. 'Feeding the city: medieval London and its agrarian hinterland', *The London Journal* **16**, 3–14.

Harvey, B. F. 1993: *Living and Dying in England, 1100–1540: The Monastic Experience* (Oxford).

Hedges, R. E., Clement, J. G., Thomas, C. D. and O'Connell T, C. 2007. 'Collagen turnover in the adult femoral mid-shaft: modeled from anthropogenic radiocarbon tracer measurements', *American Journal of Physical Anthropology* **133**, 808–816.

Mays, S. A. 1997. 'Carbon stable isotope ratios in medieval and later human skeletons from Northern England', *Journal of Archaeological Science* **24**, 561–567.

Mays, S. A., Richards, M. P. and Fuller, B. T. 2002. 'Bone stable isotope evidence for infant feeding in medieval England', *Antiquity* **76**, 654–656.

Müldner, G. and Richards, M. P. 2005. 'Fast or feast: reconstructing diet in later medieval England by stable isotope analysis', *Journal of Archaeological Science* **32**, 39–48.

Müldner, G. and Richards, M. P. 2007a. 'Diet and diversity at later medieval Fishergate: the isotopic evidence', *American Journal of Physical Anthropology* **134** (2), 162–174.

Müldner, G. and Richards, M. P. 2007b. 'Stable isotope evidence for 1500 years of human diet at the city of York, UK', *American Journal of Physical Anthropology* **133**, 682–697.

O'Connell, T. C. and Hedges, R. E. M. 1999. 'Investigations into the effect of diet on modern human hair isotopic values', *American Journal of Physical Anthropology* **108**, 409–425.

Orme, N. and Webster, M. 1995. *The English Hospital, 1070–1570* (London).

Privat, K. L., O'Connell, T. C. and Richards, M. P. 2002. 'Stable isotope analysis of human and faunal remains from the Anglo-Saxon cemetery at Berinsfield, Oxfordshire: dietary and social implications', *Journal of Archaeological Science* **29**, 779–790.

Rawcliffe, C. 1995. *Medicine and Society in Later Medieval England* (Stroud).

Richards, M. P., Mays, S. A. and Fuller, B. T. 2002. 'Stable carbon and nitrogen isotope values of bone and teeth reflect weaning age at the medieval Wharram Percy site, Yorkshire, UK', *American Journal of Physical Anthropology* **119**, 205–210.

Russell, J. C. 1959. 'Medieval Midland and northern migration to London 1100–1365', *Speculum* **34**, 641–645.

Schoeninger, M. J. and DeNiro, M. J. 1984. 'Stable nitrogen and carbon isotopic composition of bone collagen from marine and terrestrial animals', *Geochimica et Cosmochimica Acta* **48**, 625–639.

Schofield, J. 1997. 'Excavations on the site of St Nicholas Shambles, Newgate Street, City of London, 1975–9', *Transactions of the City of London and Middlesex Archaeology Society* **48**, 77–135.

Sealy, J. 2001. 'Body tissue chemistry and palaeodiet', in Brothwell, D. R. and Pollard, A. M. (ed.) *Handbook of Archaeological Science* (Chichester), 269–279.

Thomas, C. 2002. *The Archaeology of Medieval London* (Stroud).

Thomas, C., Sloane, B. and Phillpotts, C. 1997. Excavations at the Priory and Hospital of St Mary Spital, London (London).

Thrupp, S.L. 1989. *The Merchant Class of Medieval London, 1300–1500* (Ann Arbor).

Woolgar, C. M., Serjeantson, D. and Waldron, T. 2006. *Food in Medieval England: Diet and Nutrition* (Oxford).

New Temptations?
Olive, Cherry and Mulberry in Roman and Medieval Europe

Alexandra Livarda,
University of Leicester

Many influential anthropological and sociological studies have stressed that food does not simply cover people's physiological needs but has a more profound significance, both underlying and actively contributing to the fabric of social structure. Following this rationale, this short study is based on the premise that food is a social event and a tool for the construction and maintenance of social identity, and thus it can be used to infer status and social relations in the past. Within this framework, an exploration of food preferences and distribution is attempted from an archaeological perspective. The actual focus is on exotic food plants, since these are one of the most easily identifiable indicators of social context in terms of archaeobotanical data (Palmer and Van der Veen 2002). Naturally, the notion of exotic is a relative one, as the same species may have different connotations in different parts of the world and at different historical periods. This very notion constitutes the point of concern of the present research, which is part of a larger research project directed by Professor M. van der Veen at the University of Leicester. The dispersal histories of a large number of food plants, imported or newly introduced into north-west Europe between the Roman and later-medieval periods (*ca.* 100 BC–AD 1500) are examined. Here, three examples are presented to give a first indication of the overall results and of the potential value of such studies. Patterns of access to and consumption of olive (*Olea europaea* L.), cherry (*Prunus avium/cerasus* L.) and mulberry (*Morus nigra* L.) are examined, using archaeobotanical data as evidence. The aim is to illustrate the contrasting dispersal histories of these fruits, who had access to them, whether access changed over time and whether they became integrated into the local staple diet and agricultural system.

The Fruits
Olive and mulberry are not native to north-west Europe, being first introduced to the area during the Roman period. Olive (*Olea europaea* L.) is native to the Mediterranean (Zohary and Hopf 2000, 145), where it was exploited from prehistoric times, according to charcoal and seed finds (for instance Terral and Arnold-Simard 1996; Foxhall 2007, 10–13), and later became an important part of Roman agricultural and culinary traditions. Mulberry (*Morus nigra* L.) probably originates from Iran and was known to Greeks and Romans by the late first millennium BC (Vaughan and Geissler 1999, 100). It can be successfully cultivated in areas with Mediterranean and mild temperate climates (Gerasopoulos and

Roman	
Rural	lesser, nucleated, élite
Urban	major, minor
Military	extramural, intramural
Ceremonial	burial, temple/shrine
Other	industrial, shipwreck

Early medieval and medieval	
Rural	lesser, village, élite
Urban	major, minor, castle
Trading Centre	only for the EM
Religious	urban monastery, rural monastery, cemetery/burial
Other	industrial, shipwreck

Table 8.1. Site-type classification for each time period.

Stavroulakis 1997, 261). Other economic *Morus* species exist, such as *Morus alba* that arrived in southern Europe during the late Roman period (Prance and Nesbitt 2005, 346), but here only *Morus nigra*, as identified in the archaeobotanical reports, is examined. Cherry (*Prunus avium/cerasus* L.) is different in that its wild form is present in temperate Europe; current thought is, however, that the Romans introduced the domesticated form of cherry into northern Europe (Watkins 1995, 425).

Method

Secondary archaeobotanical data from several hundred excavation reports from northwest and western Europe, including the present-day countries of Belgium, Britain, Denmark, France, Germany, Luxembourg, Spain, Switzerland, and The Netherlands, were collected for the Roman to medieval periods. Information was drawn from sites that included at least one condiment, fruit, vegetable and so on, that was introduced and/or became largely exploited into parts of or the whole study area at any point during this 1600-year period. From this dataset, information on olive, cherry, and mulberry was selected for the present study.

The presence and preservation mode of these species were recorded but as waterlogging was their dominant state of preservation, only this type of data is included here. Different types of food plants usually survive in distinct preservation modes according to their various uses and the processing stages they have to go through to be prepared for consumption/usage. Fruits would not normally come in contact with fire – as opposed to cereals for example – and, therefore, carbonized fruit remains are generally few in number (for instance Willerding 1971). Comparing species with the same chances of being retrieved is imperative in order to be consistent and avoid biases. However, it should be noted that since fruits are mostly found in waterlogged conditions, which are usually typical of deep deposits, most frequently encountered in urban rather than rural contexts, some biases may exist in their social distribution. Yet since the same bias applies for all three fruits and all time periods their comparison can still provide useful insights into their patterning.

Site type	Roman	Early Medieval	Medieval
Burial	5	2	3
Temple-shrine	9	-	-
Monastery rural	-	1	12
Monastery urban	-	-	19
Military extramural	36	-	-
Military intramural	45	-	-
Military unknown	1	-	-
Rural élite	35	6	32
Rural lesser	50	12	20
Rural non élite	8	7	7
Rural nucleated/village	27	25	18
Town major	80	23	201
Town minor	29	6	107
Castle	-	-	4
Trading centre	-	12	-
Industrial site	3	-	2
Shipwreck	3	2	3
Totals	331	96	428

Table 8.2. *Number of waterlogged sites per time period.*

The three fruits are here analysed according to their chronological, social and geographical dispersal. In order to trace chronological changes all the data were categorized as Roman (100 BC–AD 500), early medieval (AD 500–950) or medieval (AD 950–1500). Closer dating of the individual sites was also recorded and will be highlighted when necessary; a more detailed chronological analysis is planned for the future. Furthermore, to monitor social access, each site was classified into broad units (Tab. 8.1); as different forms of socio-political organization were evident in the Roman and the medieval worlds, a distinct set of broad categories was employed for each time period, while acknowledging that the Roman/medieval division is artificial and varies in each region.

A 'site' refers to an excavation phase dated to one of the three noted periods; a big city such as London, may therefore be represented by several 'sites'. When more than one type of site occurred on an excavation (for instance a temple and residential area in a major town) then two records were made, one for each site type. Currently the dataset has a good number of medieval and Roman sites but the early medieval period is

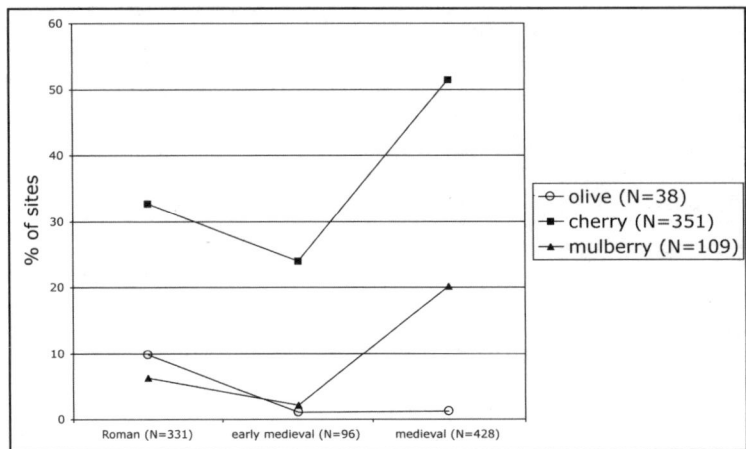

Figure 8.1. Chronological distribution of waterlogged records of olive, cherry and mulberry, indicating for each time period the proportion of sites with each fruit over the total number of sites with newly introduced food plants. N= the total number of waterlogged records. The total number of sites per time period is given on horizontal axis.

under-represented. Roman records are distributed mostly over military, urban and rural sites; the early medieval records contain slightly more rural sites; urban sites dominate the medieval records (Tab. 8.2).

The Archaeobotanical Evidence: Olive

The chronological distribution of olive (Fig. 8.1) shows that this fruit was relatively common under Rome but its occurrence dropped significantly in the following two periods. More detailed dating evidence suggests that olive was present in the study area from the early Roman period but its decline was already observed by the end of the third/beginning of the fourth century AD. Under Rome, olive is mainly associated with major towns and, to a lesser extent, military sites, while in terms of rural sites waterlogged olive evidence has been recorded only from élite contexts (Fig. 8.2).

The olive's spatial dispersal (Fig. 8.3) during this period shows that it occurs predominantly in the southern part of the study area and along the Rhine frontier. Considering that waterlogged seed assemblages are rare in the southern region, there is a bias against the recovery of fruits, the preponderance of olive highlights its strong association with this region and reflects its important role (and that of its derivatives) in everyday diet and life. This interpretation is supported by the increased production and commercialization of olives and olive oil in parts of the Mediterranean, with Baetica, Spain, being a typical example, and the widespread consumption of the fruit as attested in contemporary texts (Mattingly 1988; Brun 2003, 144–6). In the northern provinces, olive is an import and seems to be associated with military sites and major towns – London, York, Xanten, and Cologne – all of which had a strong military presence.

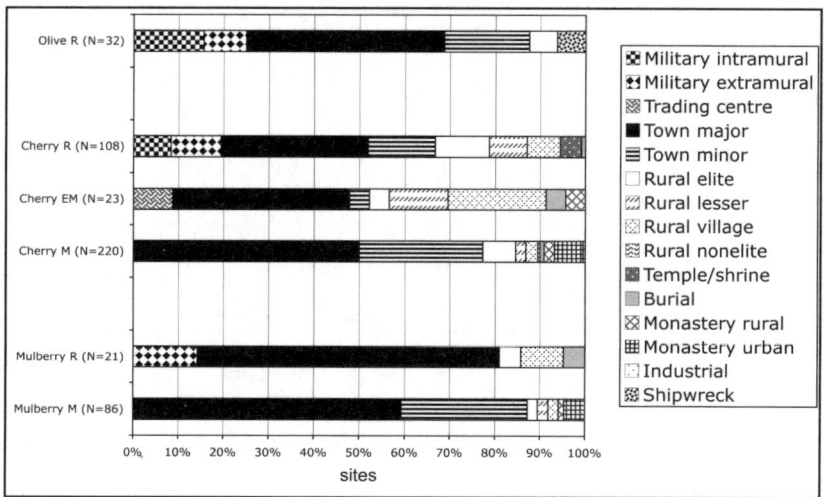

Figure 8.2. Social access to the three fruits for each period (R= Roman, EM = early medieval, M= medieval). N= the number of waterlogged records of each fruit (where N<20 no information is provided).

Overall, the evidence indicates that olive imports in the northern provinces were already in operation during the very early stages of Roman expansion, its spread being largely associated with the movement into the area of people from a different culinary tradition. Furthermore, its absence from rural non-élite sites would seem to confirm its exotic status. The occasional encounter of olive on rural élite sites may suggest a possible luxury status for the fruit but it could also mean that people inhabiting these élite sites were affiliated with Romans. The restriction of imported olives, as demonstrated by the archaeobotanical records, to relatively few sites, albeit frequently in large quantities, stands in sharp contrast with the comparatively ample ceramic evidence (amphorae) for the importation of olive oil (see Remesal Rodríguez 1998, 187, 198; Jones and Mattingly 1993, 196–7). Full consideration of this difference is outside the scope of this paper but an answer may be sought along the lines of the distinct uses of the two products. As soon as Roman control deteriorates, the evidence for olive declines drastically. On the whole, the archaeobotanical evidence shows that the olive did not become part of the staple diet in the northern part of the study area and from the third century AD onwards became a rarity. Strikingly, very few early medieval and medieval olive records exist (Tab. 8.3); those that do are associated with urban sites.

The Archaeobotanical Evidence: Cherry

Cherry was apparently common in north-west Europe throughout the study period, with a peak in the medieval phase (Fig. 8.1 and Tab. 8.3). During the Roman period cherry is present on over 30 per cent of all sites in the dataset; in the early medieval phase there is a drop in its occurrence but it is still relatively common at more than 20

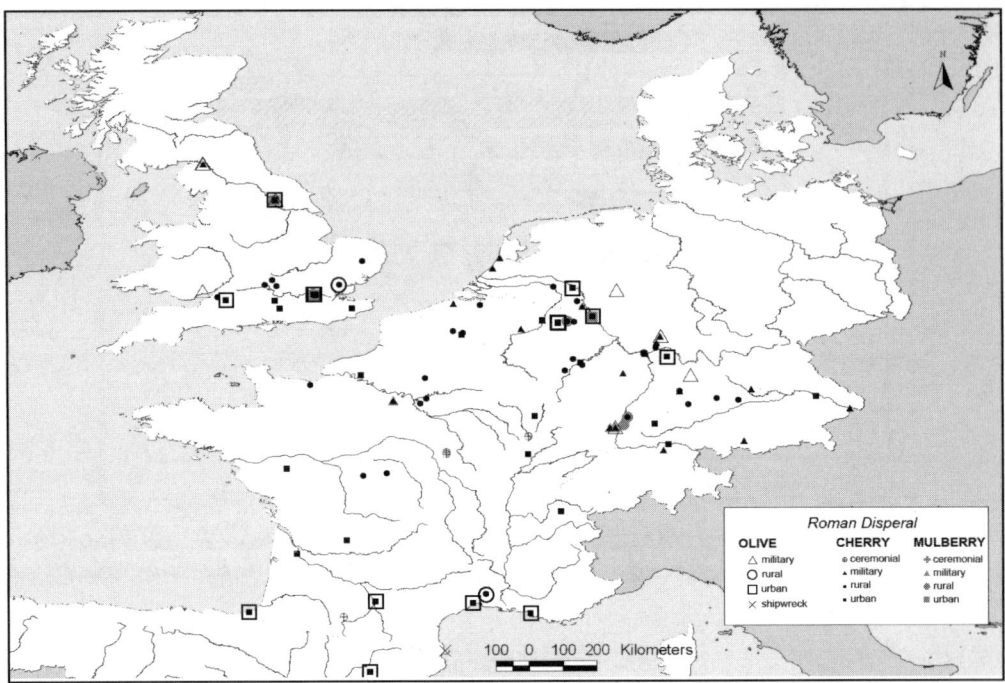

Figure 8.3. Geographical dispersal of waterlogged olive, cherry and mulberry during the Roman period. The study area is given in white.

per cent; finally, in the medieval period the occurrence of cherry increases to more than 50 per cent of all sites. Closer dating shows that cherry was already present during the early stages of Roman occupation and continued to be quite prominent through the late Roman period; following a relative decline, it became significant again from the twelfth century onwards.

Its social dispersal (Fig. 8.2) shows how cherry is found mainly on Roman urban, followed by rural and military sites, with a roughly equal proportion of rural élite and non-élite contexts. In the early medieval period it is associated principally with rural non-élite sites and major towns; in the Middle Ages a strong urban association is discerned, while within the rural category cherry is present primarily on élite sites. However, the fact that the medieval data derive largely from urban sites may skew the results, hiding the trends for other site types. This possibility was examined by

	Roman	Early Medieval	Medieval	Total
Olive	32	1	5	38
Cherry	108	23	220	351
Mulberry	21	2	86	109

Table 8.3. Number of waterlogged records per time period.

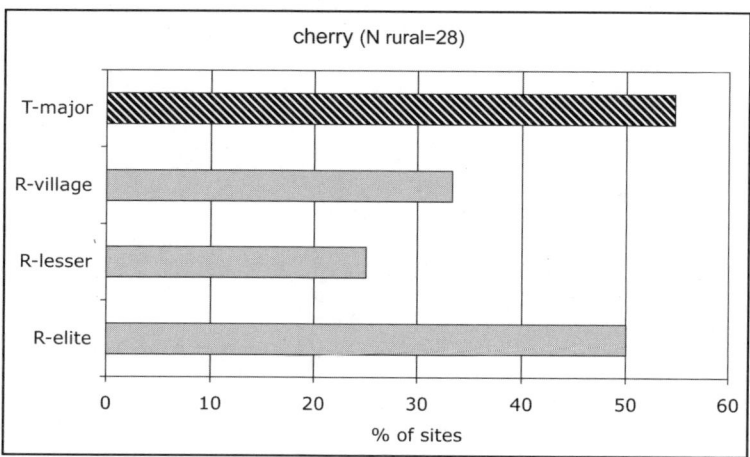

Figure 8.4. Proportion of all rural site types and major towns with waterlogged cherry during the medieval period, expressed as a percentage of their total number in the dataset (T = town, R = rural). N rural = the absolute number of all medieval rural sites where cherry occurs.

employing a different analytical approach: the proportion of the various rural site types with waterlogged cherry as a percentage of the total number of each rural site type in the dataset for the medieval period was calculated, and adding the major town data for comparison (Fig. 8.4). This indicates that cherry has indeed some rural association, being found on half of the rural élite sites – a comparable proportion to its presence in major towns – and on a substantial proportion of all villages and lesser sites recorded.

The geographical dispersal of this fruit during the Roman period (Fig. 8.3) illustrates its presence on a variety of sites along and within the *limes*. In Britain, most evidence comes from the south and south-east, but find-spots also occur on military sites and in York. In the early medieval phase there is a significant change: the few cherry records cluster in the northern and north-eastern parts of the study area, with the majority of the rural sites being confined towards the western and southern margins of its distribution (Fig. 8.5). The picture changes again in the medieval period (Fig. 8.6) when cherry is found in nearly every part of the study area. A strong urban association is evident, whereas rural sites with cherry can be identified mostly in central-southern modern-day France and The Netherlands.

Cherry was, therefore, relatively widespread in the study area from the early stages of the Roman conquest through to the medieval period. Although cherries were collected from the wild during prehistory, their systematic exploitation by grafting did not occur in the northern provinces until introduced by the Romans (Bakels and Jacomet 2003, 554–5), which is also supported by the lower numbers of cherry seeds and fruits retrieved from pre-Roman northern contexts (for example Pollmann *et al.* 2005, 1471). This familiarity with the consumption of cherry may have been the trigger

Olive, Cherry and Mulberry in Roman and Medieval Europe

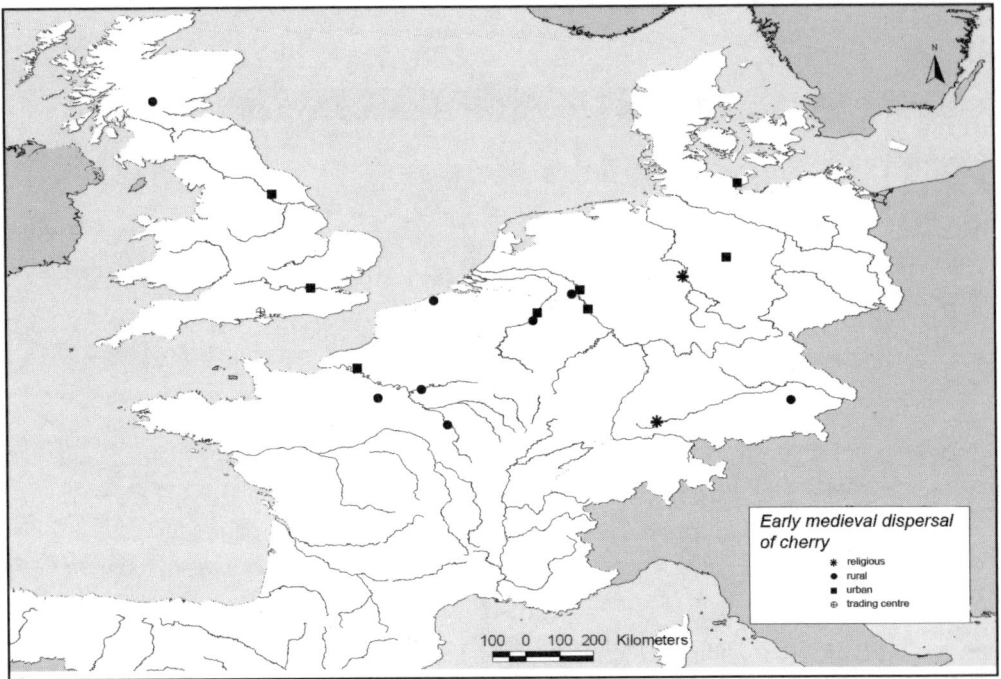

Figure 8.5. Geographical dispersal of waterlogged cherry during the early medieval period. The study area is given in white

for the adoption of the new exploitation methods by local people and the consequent increased incorporation of cherry into the diet. Its widespread diffusion and its presence on quite a few Roman rural sites, many of which are élite, may indicate its cultivation and extensive use within the framework of a changing culinary culture. Evidence from early medieval villages and individual farmsteads may suggest the continuation of its importance and its expansion towards the north-east. Later on, from the twelfth century, the expansion of urbanism, urban markets, and the improvement of fruit-tending techniques can provide an explanation for the increased access to cherry.

Overall, the archaeobotanical data suggest that systematic exploitation of cherry increased with the Romans from the early stages of their expansion to the north. Cherry continued to be used throughout the study period by various sectors of society and by the late Middle Ages it was dispersed across some of the northernmost parts of Europe.

The Archaeobotanical Evidence: Mulberry

In contrast to the other two fruits, mulberry is relatively rare in the Roman period. A further drop in its occurrence, albeit slight, can be observed during the early medieval phase and only later in the medieval period does its occurrence increase significantly (Fig. 8.1). Its limited Roman evidence is mainly restricted to major towns (Fig. 8.2) while the early medieval data are particularly poor (Tab. 8.3) deriving merely from a

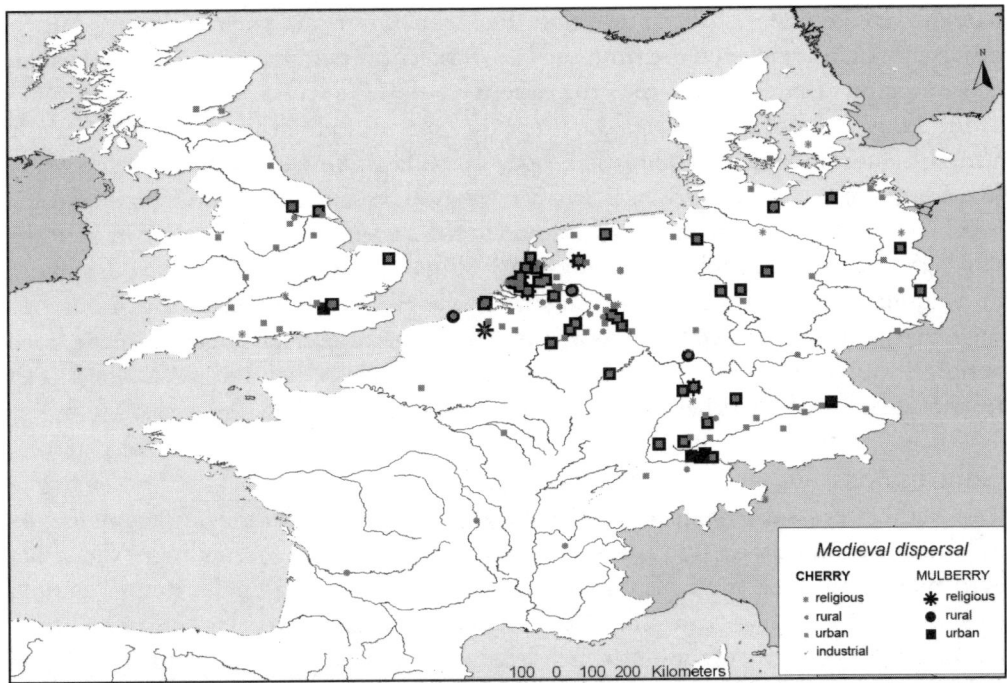

Figure 8.6. Geographical dispersal of waterlogged cherry and mulberry during the medieval period. The study area is given in white.

major town and a rural lesser site. In the medieval period a strong urban association becomes apparent with the fruit being particularly rare on all types of rural sites (Fig. 8.2), having been recorded only on six of them. The geographical dispersal of mulberry further indicates its presence at a few selected Roman sites (Fig. 8.3), and a shift in its medieval occurrences towards the north-east (Fig. 8.6).

Significantly, mulberry needs to be fully ripe before it is consumed and is particularly prone to damage (Cool 2006, 122). Cool thus suggests that instances of mulberry in Roman Britain are indicative of the introduction of the tree rather than the fruit; alternatively it could be anticipated that they were imported as dried fruits. Whatever the form of introduction, mulberry was a rare Roman food plant. In reality almost all of its finds are associated with London, outside of which it is found only on two urban sites, one in York and another in Cologne. Even the mulberry record for burials (Fig. 8.2) originates from the Eastern cemetery in London. The few rural sites are all on the Continent. Interestingly, the two rural nucleated sites are situated near the Rhine, in close proximity to two military sites. The third rural site, this time élite, is also located near the Rhine and the *Colonia* of Cologne. Thus, some connection with the Roman military can be postulated but its wide availability in London may hint at mulberry's luxury status in the context of this particular urban Roman society.

In the early medieval period, there are just two records for mulberry in the northern part of the Continent. It becomes more frequent during the twelfth century but its occurrence increases even more from the late fourteenth century onwards. The apparent concentration of mulberry towards the eastern coast of England and the north-east part of the study area possibly reflects the intensification of trade in the north, particularly after the emergence of the Hanseatic League at the beginning of the thirteenth century (see Karg 2007). It may also be linked to the growth of the German Empire, which became the strongest state in Christendom after the twelfth century and controlled the northern trade routes. Mulberry is once again ubiquitous in London but it is also found in multiple contexts in other major towns of the period. Its absence from rural sites suggests that it was not widely adopted by all sectors of society. By the late medieval period it was not yet an integral part of northern European diet; instead mulberry can be considered a largely urban phenomenon, possibly an exotic garden tree.

Conclusions

This study gives some insights into the factors underlying the changes and complexities of human diet in historic times. The examples of olive, cherry, and mulberry show that even though all three fruits were available from the beginning of the Roman period, each followed a distinct path. The familiarity of cherry and its ecological suitability to temperate Europe led very soon to the dispersal of the species in all sectors of society, to become part of the northern European environment and diet. In contrast, olive and mulberry were true exotics in the sense that neither of the two seems to have been integrated into the local agricultural regimes of north-west Europe. Olive, with a strong association with Mediterranean customs, was introduced during the Roman period to the north-western provinces, possibly owing to army demands, and became a luxury item for part of the population. It is rather rare, considering its strong association with Roman cuisine and in contrast to the relative ubiquity of olive oil. Mulberry was a rare Roman exotic fruit not related to the standard Roman military diet but probably employed as a means of social differentiation, especially in London and a few sites in the Rhine area. It was possibly cultivated in Europe by the medieval period, but its remains derive primarily from towns, perhaps suggesting it remained a luxury, used as a means of social distinction.

The historical dispersal of the fruits under consideration highlights a changing culinary culture and the transient nature of the status of the various species, while underlining the importance of the interplay between environmental, social and economic parameters in the shaping of north-western Europe. Moreover, this contextual analysis contributes further evidence to indicate the complexities of the interaction between different peoples in different historical contexts. The incorporation of archaeobotanical data on more species and a further refined temporal and social dispersal analysis hold the potential to shed more light and provide more fascinating insights into the shaping of Europe as we know it.

Olive, Cherry and Mulberry in Roman and Medieval Europe

Acknowledgements

This research, being part of my PhD thesis, was funded by Prof. Van der Veen's NERC project on 'Long-Distance Trade and Agricultural Development', The Alexander S. Onassis Public Benefit Foundation and The A.G. Leventis Foundation. Special thanks go to Prof. M. van der Veen and Dr N. Christie for their comments and constant support. This research would not have been realised without the invaluable collaboration of the following people: Natàlia Alonso, Almuth Alsleben, Laurent Bouby, Anne Bouchette, Otto Brinkkemper, Christoph Brombacher, Ramon Buxó, Gill Campbell, Wendy Carruthers, Astrid Caseldine, Mike Charles, Marina Ciaraldi, Brigitte Cooremans, Anne Davies, Frédérique Durand, John Giorgi, James Greig, Allan Hall, Alistair Hill, Tim Holden, Jacqui Huntley, Stefanie Jacomet, Simon James, Sabine Karg, Dimitris Kourkoulis, Margarethe König, Angela Kreuz, Helmut Kroll, Christine Laurent, Philippe Marinval, Veronique Matterne, David Mattingly, Lieselotte Meersschaert, Jennifer Miller, Lisa Moffett, Nevin Moledina, Angela Monckton, Jacob Morales, Alex Moseley, Peter Murphy, Reinder Neef, Ruth Pelling, Leonor Peña-Chocarro, Bénédicte Pradat, David Earle Robinson, Mark Robinson, Manfred Rösch, Marie-Pierre Ruas, Hans-Peter Stika, Vanessa Straker, Jeremy Taylor, Scott Timpany, Patricia Vandorpe, Julian Wiethold and Lydia Zapata.

References

Bakels, C. and Jacomet, S. 2003. 'Access to luxury foods in central Europe during the Roman period: the archaeobotanical evidence', *World Archaeology* **34** (3), 542–557.

Brun, J-P. 2003. *Le Vin et l'Huile dans la Méditerranée Antique: Viticulture, Oléiculture et Procédés de Transformation* (Paris).

Cool, H. E. M. 2006. *Eating and Drinking in Roman Britain* (Cambridge).

Foxhall, L. 2007. *Olive Cultivation in Ancient Greece: Seeking the Ancient Economy* (Oxford).

Gerasopoulos, D. and Stavroulakis, G. 1997. 'Quality characteristics of four mulberry (*Morus* sp) cultivars in the area of Chania, Greece', *Journal of the Science of Food and Agriculture* **73** (2), 261–264.

Jones, B. and Mattingly, D. 1993. *An Atlas of Roman Britain* (Oxford).

Karg, S. 2007 (ed.). *Medieval Food Traditions in Northern Europe* (Copenhagen).

Mattingly, D. J. 1988. 'Oil for export? A comparison of Libyan, Spanish and Tunisian olive oil production in the Roman Empire', *Journal of Roman Archaeology* **1**, 33–56.

Palmer, C. and Veen, M. van der 2002. 'Archaeobotany and the social context of food', *Acta Palaeobotanica* **42** (2), 195–202.

Pollmann, B, Jacomet, S. and Schlumbaum, A. 2005. 'Morphological and genetic studies of waterlogged *Prunus* species from the Roman *vicus Tasgetium* (Eschenz, Switzerland)', *Journal of Archaeological Science* **32** (10), 1471–1480.

Prance, G. and Nesbitt, M. 2005 (eds.). *The Cultural History of Plants* (London).

Remesal Rodríguez, J. 1998. 'Baetican olive oil and the Roman economy', in Keay, S. (ed.) *The Archaeology of Early Roman Baetica* (Portsmouth, Rhode Island), 183–199.

Terral, J-F. and Arnold-Simard, G. 1996. 'Beginnings of olive cultivation in Eastern Spain in relation to Holocene bioclimatic changes', *Quaternary Research* **46**, 176–185.

Vaughan, J. G. and Geissler, C. A. 1999. *The New Oxford Book of Food Plants* (Oxford).

Watkins, R. 1995. 'Cherry, plum, peach, apricot and almond', in Smartt, J. and Simmonds, N. W. (eds) *Evolution of Crop Plants*. 2nd edition (Harlow), 423–428.

Willerding, U. 1971. 'Methodische Probleme bei der Untersuchng und Auswertung von Pflanzenfunden in vor- und frühgeschichtlichen Siedlungen', *Nachrichten aus Niedersachsens Urgeschichte* **40**, 180–198.

Zohary, D. and Hopf, M. 2000. *Domestication of Plants in the Old World* (Oxford).

Gathered Food Plants at Dutch Mesolithic and Neolithic Wetland Sites

Welmoed Out,
Leiden University

Introduction

Today, acculturation is considered a key process in neolithization of many regions at the fringe of north-west Europe (Barker 2006, 364-381). Acculturation can be characterized as a mosaic of local processes that influenced ideology, material culture and subsistence. For Britain and Ireland it has been argued that ideology and material culture changed quickly, while subsistence practices changed more gradually (Thomas 1999). However, Rowley-Conwy (2004) has suggested that the incorporation of domestic animals and crop plants may actually have occurred fairly rapidly in many parts of north-west Europe. Unfortunately, the rate of incorporation of crop plants into subsistence strategies is difficult to reconstruct in detail because quantitative analysis of the ratio of crop plants to gathered plants is hampered by differential representation and recovery (see Rowley-Conwy 2004).

There is substantial evidence that the neolithization of the Lower Rhine area was a gradual acculturation process, characterized by the introduction of pottery at *ca.* 5000 BC, the introduction of domestic animals at *ca.* 4700 BC and the introduction of crop plants around *ca.* 4200 BC. At least until the end of the Middle Neolithic (at 3400/3300 BC), subsistence was based on a combination of hunting, gathering, fishing, fowling and agriculture, representing an extended broad-spectrum economy. Only in the Late Neolithic did the economy become based on agriculture more firmly (Louwe Kooijmans 2007; Raemaekers 1999). From the point of their introduction, cereals are found in domestic deposits at almost all Dutch wetland sites (Out in press), suggesting their rapid incorporation into daily life. The precise economic importance of crop plants is, however, difficult to assess because simple counts of archaeological crop remains provide insufficient information. Rather than studying the neolithization process by focussing on crop plants, this paper considers the evidence from gathered food plants. The study is based on data from Dutch wetland sites dating to *ca.* 5500–3400 BC, which corresponds with the Late Mesolithic, the Early/Middle Neolithic Swifterbant Culture (4900–3400 BC) and the Middle Neolithic Hazendonk Group in the central part of the Netherlands (3800–3400 BC). At the wetland sites, preservation of organic material is generally good due to continuous sedimentation under waterlogged conditions.

Analysis of gathered food plants from Mesolithic/Neolithic Dutch wetland sites is not new but a critical overview of indications for their consumption is lacking. This

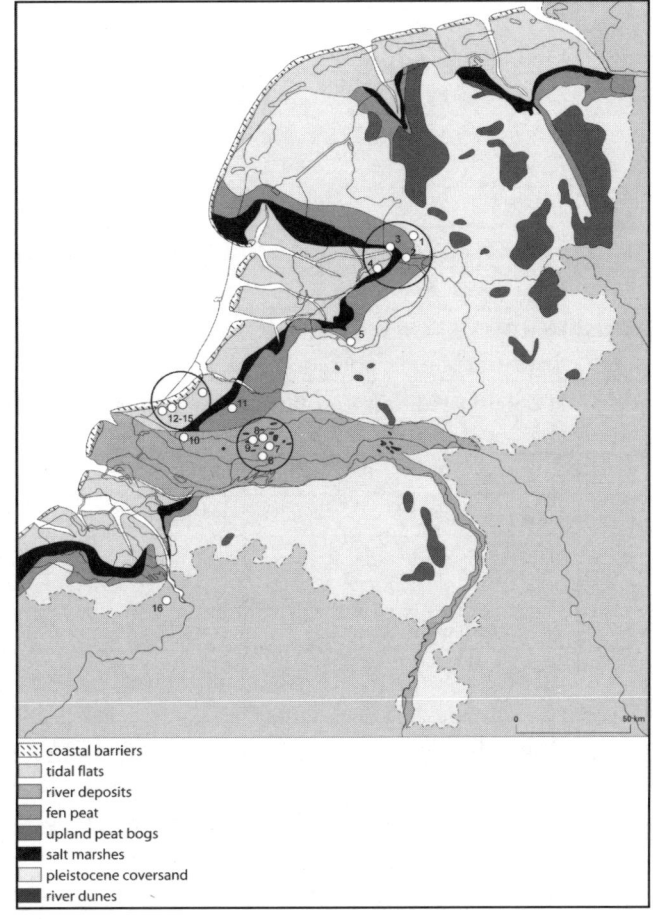

Figure 9.1. Palaeogeographic map of the Netherlands at 4200 cal BC (after Louwe Kooijmans 2007), with the location of the sites included in the presented analysis. Table 1 gives the names of the sites. The three main regions are indicated with circles.

paper is based on data synthesized from publications and grey literature available at the time of writing. It will investigate which taxa were probably consumed on a considerable scale; whether it is possible to discern differences between various regions; and whether temporal changes related to the neolithization process can be discerned. Some attention is paid to food preparation and consumption. A comparison is finally made with the scarce information from Dutch and Belgian dryland sites.

Materials and Methods

Figure 9.1 and table 9.1 show the sites included in the study, plotted on a palaeogeographic map of the Netherlands (*ca.* 4200 BC). Three main regions can be discerned with a concentration of sites: the northern region, the southern river area and the coastal region. The number and type of samples collected at each site is highly variable, depending on the research methods and scale of excavation. Common sample contexts are refuse layers, pits, unlined wells and hearths.

Gathered Food Plants at Dutch Wetland Sites

No.	Site	Occupation (yrs BC)	Reference
1	Schokland-P14	4900–3300	Gehasse 1995
2	Schokland-Zuiderhaven-E170	3950–3700	Gehasse 1995; Luijten 1987
3	Urk-E4	7000–3500	Peters and Peeters 2001
4	Swifterbant-S3	4400–4100	Van Zeist and Palfenier-Vegter 1981
5	Hoge Vaart-A27	6600–4150	Visser *et al.* 2001
6	Hardinxveld-Giessendam De Bruin	5500–4550	Bakels *et al.* 2001
	Hardinxveld-Giessendam Polderweg	5500–5000	Bakels and Van Buerden 2001
7	Brandwijk-Kerkhof	4600–3600	Out 2008
8	Hazendonk	4020–3610	Bakels and Kuijper unpublished data
9	Streefkerk-Zijdeweg	5220–5100	Verbruggen and Kuijper unpublished data
10	Rotterdam-Randstadrail	5630–5380	Guiran and Brinkkemper 2007
11	Bergschenhoek	4300–4100	Casparie, Bakels and Kuijper unpublished data
12	Wateringen-4	3625–3400	Raemaekers *et al.* 1997
13	Schipluiden	3630–3380	Kubiak-Martens 2006a
14	Rijswijk-A4	Middle Neolithic	Bakels and Kuijper unpublished data
15	Rijswijk-Ypenburg	3860–3435	Koot and Van der Have 2001; Van Haaster 2001
16	Doel Deurganckdok-sector B	<3960–3710	Bastiaens *et al.* 2005

Table 9.1. *The sites included in the study, with information on the occupation period and reference. The occupation dates only show occupation during the Late Mesolithic until the Middle Neolithic but not later occupation.*

The analysis of gathered food plants is primarily based on seeds (in the broadest sense of the word) and tubers, since these are usually the best preserved. In order to identify which taxa probably played an important role in the diet, initial investigation focused on the plants most likely to have been handled by people. The following criteria were considered as indicative for handling/use by people (see Dietsch 1996): presence of seeds in carbonized state; presence of carbonized seeds in a high or moderate frequency; presence of carbonized seeds in hearths; presence of seeds in anthropogenic concentrations (a pure concentration containing a quantity of seeds that can not be explained by non-human processes such as absence of seed transport or collection by animals); occurrence of seeds in an anthropogenic spatial distribution; and indications of use by use-wear analysis and phytolith analysis from artefacts. This analysis resulted in a list of probably used plants including food plants. In order to identify the food plants in this group, the edibility, energy value and the storage suitability of the relevant seeds was taken into account (based on a variety of archaeobotanical sources). Scarce evidence of consumption from plant remains in food crusts and coprolites was also considered.

Tubers, including roots and bulbs, form a separate category. They are usually preserved in a carbonized state and when recovered, especially from hearths, it is often assumed that they represent food. However, it is possible that tubers were carbonized inadvertently, for instance if they grew naturally in the soil near the hearth. Identification of tubers also depends on attention paid to recovery, and the skills and equipment of individual researchers. For all these reasons it is difficult to assess the strength of the evidence of consumption.

Food Plants

Table 9.2 summarizes the evidence of gathered-plant consumption, additionally giving information on the presence of cereals at the sites in order to highlight this aspect of neolithization. The data suggest that the hazel-nut (*Corylus avellana*) and water chestnut (*Trapa natans*) probably functioned as staple foods, since these taxa meet many criteria for use and consumption, provide high levels of energy and can be stored easily. Interestingly, there is one site in the river area (Streefkerk-Zijdeweg, not shown in table 9.2) that contains high frequencies of water chestnut remains, suggesting that people there were collecting and processing them on a considerable scale (M. Verbruggen, pers. comm.). The site was only investigated by coring and it is not yet possible to make final conclusions. The fruits of hawthorn (*Crataegus monogyna*), crab apple (*Malus sylvestris*) and sloe (*Prunus spinosa*) were probably also consumed in great numbers: all three species are regularly found in carbonized state, are very rich in energy and may have been stored after drying.

Some intermediate evidence of plant use and consumption is available for the fruits of dogwood (*Cornus sanguinea*), oak (*Quercus* sp.), blackberry (*Rubus fruticosus*), raspberry (*Rubus idaeus*), dewberry (*Rubus caesius*), rose (*Rosa* sp.), white water lily (*Nymphaea alba*) and yellow water lily (*Nuphar lutea*), but the precise importance and function of some of these taxa is not fully understood. For instance, the function and edibility of dogwood fruits is a subject of debate (Dietsch 1996, 91). Rose hips and the berries (*Rubus* sp.) are edible and supply a considerable amount of energy, but the indications for their use and consumption are restricted. This may be for several reasons: for instance these taxa produce no waste products (e.g. nut scales), their processing does not require the use of fire and so they are unlikely to form part of the charred assemblages on which this analysis focuses. Seeds and tubers from the white and yellow water lily may have been consumed, but carbonized tubers of these species have not

Gathered Food Plants at Dutch Wetland Sites

	Schokland-P14	Schokland-Zuiderhaven-E170	Urk-E4	Swifterbant-S3	Abundance	HG De Bruin	HG Polderweg	Brandwijk-Kerkhof	Hazendonk	Abundance
Region			North					South		
Cereals	-/+	+	-/+	+		-	-	-/+	+	
Corylus avellana	c,w	c,w	c,w	c,w	2	c,w	c,w	c,w	c,w	3
Crataegus monogyna			c	c,w	1	c,w	w	w	c,w	2
Malus sylvestris			c	c,w	1	c	c,w	w	c,w	2
Prunus spinosa							w	w	c,w	2
Trapa natana	c				1	c,w	c,w	c,w	c	2
Cornus sanguinea				w		c,w	w	c,w	c,w	2
Quercus sp.	c,w				1	c,w	w	w	c,w	3
Nuphar lutea		w			1	w	w	w	w	2
Nymphaea alba		w		w	1			c,w	c,w	2
Rosa sp.				w	1	w	w			1
Rubus sp.	c	w			1					
Rubus caesius						w	w		w	1
Rubus fruticosus	w		w	w	2			w	c,w	2
Rubus idaeus										
Sambucus nigra							w		w	2
Galium aparine		w	c	c	2	c,w		c,w	c,w	2
Juniperus communis										
Prunus padus						w				1
Pyrus pyraster										
cf. *Ribes* sp.						w				1
Viburnum opulus						w	w	w	c,w	2

Table 9.2. Summarized data from the studied sites by region on presence of a selection of potential food plants, combined with indications for consumption and information on edibility, energy and suitability for storage: c = carbonized, w = waterlogged. Cereals: - = absent; + = present; -/+ = present during late phases only. 'Abundance' gives abundance of macroremains from a taxon in a region: 1 = scarce; 2 = more or less common; 3 = very common. Indications for consumption: a = presence of carbonized seeds in a high or

Gathered Food Plants at Dutch Wetland Sites

Rijswijk-Ypenburg	Wateringen-4	Schipluiden	Rijswijk-A4	Abundance	Hoge Vaart-A27	Rotterdam-Randstadrail	Bergschenhoek	Doel Deurganckdok-sector B	a	b	c	d	Energy	Edibility	Storage	Evidence
\multicolumn{5}{c}{Coastal}													
+	+	+	+		-	-	-	+								
w	c	c,w	c	1	c	c,w		c	++	+	+	+	++	+	+	+
		c,w		1				c	+	+/-			+	+	+	+
w	c,w	c,w	w	3	c,w	cf.w	w	c		+			+	+	+	+
c,w	c,w	c,w	w	3			w	c	+	+	+	+	+	+	+	+
						c,w			+	+/-		+	++	+	+	+
	w	c,w	w	1		c,w		c,w	+	+/-	?		+	+/-	+	+/-
					c	c	w			+		+	++	+	+	+/-
						c,w	w	w					+	+	?	+/-
						c,w	w	w					+	+	?	+/-
	c	c,w	w	2									+	+	+	+/-
	w	w	w	2		w							+/-	+	+/-	+/-
w		w	w	2							?		+/-	+	+/-	+/-
w				1	c					+/-			+/-	+	+/-	+/-
w	w	w	w	2									+/-	+	+/-	+/-
	c	c,w	c	2	c	c,w		c	+	+			?	?	?	+/-
		w		1									+/-	+/-	+	-
													?	+	+	-
w				1									+	+	+	-
													+/-	+	-	-
													?	-	?	-

moderate frequency at many sites (++) or at two sites (+); b = taxa from which carbonized seeds have been found in hearths at a minimum of two sites (+) or at a single site (+/-); c = occurrence of seeds in anthropogenic concentrations; d = occurrence of seeds in a anthropogenic spatial distribution. Energy, edibility, storage: ++ = high; + = high/good; +/- = moderate; - = low/poor; ? = questionable/unknown. 'Evidence' gives the overall judgement on consumption of taxa. The data on Quercus do not include cupules.

yet been identified. Acorns are well known as food plants from other parts of the world but the indications for their use and consumption at Neolithic Dutch wetland sites are restricted, a situation apparently comparable to that for Late Mesolithic and Early/Middle Neolithic Scandinavia (Larsson 1990; though see Robinson 2007, 363). The status of acorns as food plants is complicated because their remains might equally represent wood-working waste or the burning of wood as fuel, as indicated by finds of juvenile nuts and cupules. Evidence of the consumption of acorns does, however, increase considerably in the Late Neolithic, as was found at the coastal site of Aartswoud (Pals 1984). Overall, the spectrum of commonly gathered food plants from this study is comparable to the spectra from other sites of the north-west European Mesolithic and Neolithic (Dietsch 1996; Jones and Rowley-Conwy 2007; Kroll 2007; Robinson 2007).

In addition to the plants discussed above, there are many more taxa that were probably consumed but for which the evidence is poor; such as for elder (*Sambucus nigra*), wild pear (*Pyrus pyraster*) for which only a single carbonized seed is known (Koot and Van der Have 2001), and juniper (*Juniperus communis*) that may have been used to flavour food. An example that stresses the bias of the dataset is the human or dog coprolite from Schipluiden that contained pollen of sea buckthorn (*Hippophae* sp.), elder (*Sambucus* sp.), bittersweet (*Solanum dulcamara*) and large grasses, possibly indicating that people consumed these taxa (Bakels 2006, 314).

As table 9.2 shows, evidence of the consumption of herbs is under-represented, probably because these plants would have been eaten as green leaves before the season of seed production and so they are difficult to trace. One exception is cleavers (*Galium aparine*) for which there is considerable evidence of its use, also at sites without cereals. Its function is unfortunately not clear, although some scholars suggest that it may have been used as a kind of coffee (Visser *et al.* 2001, 37). There is also evidence of the consumption of orache/annual seeblite (*Atriplex* sp./*Suaeda maritima*) since their seeds were recovered from food residues preserved on pottery (Kubiak-Martens 2006a, 350–351). Phytolith analysis additionally demonstrated the presence of phytoliths of wild grasses (Panicoids) on a quern stone found at Schipluiden, suggesting that they too may have been eaten (Van Gijn and Houkes 2006). These types of evidence – food residues and phytoliths – are unfortunately still scarce and need more attention in future research, the same being true of starch grains.

Tubers identified at the studied sites are lesser celandine (*Ranunculus ficaria*), onion (*Allium* sp.), sea club-rush (*Bolboschoenus maritimus*) and sea beet (*Beta vulgaris* ssp. *maritimus*). Of these, considerable evidence of consumption has been found only for lesser celandine, the bulbs of which have been found at several sites and also in hearths, mostly in the southern region and close to Rotterdam (e.g. Guiran and Brinkkemper 2007). The other tubers were found exclusively at Schipluiden, outside hearths (Kubiak-Martens 2006b).

Differences Between the Regions

There are some differences in the spectrum of gathered food plants between the three main wetland regions. In the coastal region, there is much evidence of consumption of fruits from dune shrub vegetation, such as sloe berries and crab apples, and less evidence of consumption of some deciduous woodland taxa, such as acorns and hazelnuts. The spectrum of probable plant foods in the river area is highly diverse, with relatively good indications for water chestnut consumption. In the northern region indications for presence and consumption of dogwood, hawthorn, crab apple, sloe, acorns, elder and water chestnut are scarce compared to the two other regions. This may indicate differences in the natural vegetation and/or in the food habits of the northern region; alternatively, it could simply reflect differences in research methods, taphonomy, preservation or sample size. Certainly, with the exception of Swifterbant-S3, the number of samples, identified macroremains and the number of carbonized taxa are relatively small from sites in the northern region. However, results from new excavations at Swifterbant show no finds of dogwood, sloe, acorns, elder and water chestnut, thus confirming their scarcity in the region (R. T. J. Cappers, pers. comm., Groningen Institute of Archaeology). As in earlier excavations at Swifterbant, the new research programme has yielded finds of hawthorn and crab apple/wild pear. These taxa have also been found in carbonized state at Urk-E4, perhaps indicating that they were common in the northern region.

Overall, differences in the spectrum of gathered food plants between the regions can be related primarily to differences in the natural vegetation. In the coastal dunes, dune shrub vegetation dominated the landscape (e.g. Louwe Kooijmans and Jongste 2006). In the river area, the vegetation consisted of varied deciduous woodland, alder carr and marsh vegetation (Van der Woude 1983). In the northern region, a combination of woodland, alder carr and marshes was present (Van Zeist and Palfenier-Vegter 1981), although it seems that the diversity of taxa may have been relatively small. That said, the differences between the regions may also reflect regional food and/or food preparation preferences. Interestingly, analysis of pottery and flint characteristics indicates that several cultural subgroups were present in the Dutch wetlands, whose geographical distribution shows similarities to the regions distinguished here (Raemaekers 1999). Nevertheless, it remains difficult to separate cultural factors from the effects of natural taxa availability.

Changes Through Time in Relation to the Neolithization Process

This analysis, which focuses on the presence of gathered food plants and evidence of consumption, is not able to reconstruct the importance of gathered plants versus crop plants during the Neolithic, or changes in the importance of gathered plants during neolithization. Data from the presented sites nevertheless allow identification of possible changes in the assemblage of gathered food plants during the neolithization process. The data show that the spectrum of probable gathered food plants was remarkably stable from the Late Mesolithic until the end of Middle Neolithic at Dutch wetland sites. The introduction of cultivated plans did not result in major changes in the composition of the plant diet, and it appears that crop plants were just added to the broad spectrum of food plants. This continuity corresponds very well with the gradual character of the neolithization process in the Dutch wetlands. Continuation of gathering of food plants during the Neolithic is also known from other north-west European Neolithic cultures (e.g. Dietsch 1996; Robinson 2000, 89; 2007, 369; Stevens 2007, 384).

It is only during the Late Neolithic that data for the Dutch wetlands indicate a change, such as the decreased frequency of water chestnut and increased representation of acorns. The decline in water chestnut may be related to temperature, since this is an indicator species of the Atlantic climatic optimum, which in the Netherlands ended *ca.* 3800 BC. There are several possible reasons for the increased importance of acorns. For instance, acorns may initially have had an important role as animal fodder, to become a human food source only later. During the Late Neolithic when the role of cereals had possibly become larger, acorns may have been adopted as a 'famine food' during years of poor cereal harvests. Equally, their increased representation could represent changes in cereal preparation methods (from removal of the tannins based on a method that did not involve roasting to a method that did include roasting; see De Hingh 2000, 200–202). Other possibilities also exist and more research is required if the situation is to be understood.

Preparation and Consumption

Although relevant data are scarce there are a few points that can be made about the preparation and consumption of gathered plant foods. First, inter-regional differences in the plant food spectrum suggest that people consumed those taxa that were locally available to them; there is no evidence that gathered plants were imported from other ecological zones. Second, because the analysis presented above is based on data from archaeological sites, in particular refuse layers, the results reflect domestic preparation and consumption. As such, off-site preparation and consumption will be underrepresented, especially the consumption of fruits and berries that may have been eaten on-the-hoof (e.g. *Hippophae* sp., *Rubus* sp., *Rosa* sp. and *Sambucus nigra*). Third, there is some information concerning shared preparation and/or consumption. At the Mesolithic site Hoge Vaart, for instance, the spatial distribution of hazel-nuts suggested that groups of people who shared a hearth also shared plant food (Visser *et al.* 2001). At Schipluiden, the spatial distribution of plant waste indicated that plant foods were prepared and/or consumed at the household level (Kubiak-Martens 2006a, 329). Finally, the combined data of all sites show evidence of various preparation methods, such as steeping, cooking, roasting and drying (e.g. Kubiak-Martens 2006a; Van Gijn and Houkes 2006). Use-wear analysis has additionally indicated grinding of oil-rich seeds, which possibly concerns hazel-nut, water chestnut or dogwood (Van Gijn *et al.* 2001, 177).

Comparison with Dryland Sites

Compared to the wetlands, evidence of consumption of gathered plants is restricted at Dutch Mesolithic and Neolithic dryland sites because preservation of organic material is very poor at these locations. Hazel-nut shells, which preserve well and are easy to retrieve (Jones and Rowley-Conwy 2007), are most frequently recovered from dryland sites. Other finds of carbonized plant taxa that may represent food are known from approximately ten Dutch and Belgian sites located in the middle of the dry sand regions. This small sample size does not allow a representative overview on gathered plant foods; however, it does demonstrate that data can be obtained for these regions and that archaeobotanists should attempt to retrieve plant remains other than hazel-nut shells whenever preservation allows.

Tubers from dryland sites have been analysed from Mesolithic hearths in the northern part of the Netherlands (Perry 1999, 2002). Identifications include tubers of bulrush (*Scirpus* sp.), cattail (*Typha* sp.), horsetail (*Equisetum* sp.), sea beet (*Beta vulgaris* ssp. *maritima*), male fern (*Dryopteris filix-mas*), heather (*Calluna vulgaris*) and aster family (Asteraceae). The first five taxa are well known for their edible tubers and may indeed represent food sources.

Conclusions

Analysis of gathered food plants from Dutch wetland sites belonging to the Late Mesolithic, Swifterbant Culture and Hazendonk Group indicates that the spectrum remained relatively stable during 5500–3400 BC This corresponds to the idea of the extended broad-spectrum economy of the relevant cultural groups and the gradual character of the neolithization process in the Dutch wetlands. Comparison of the different wetland regions shows some differences in the spectrum of gathered plants that can primarily be related to differences in the natural vegetation. The dataset gives some scarce evidence on preparation and consumption. The contrast to dryland regions is large, mainly due to differences in preservation conditions.

Acknowledgements

This paper is part of the project 'The harvest of Malta: from forager to farmer', conducted by Leiden University Leiden and financed by NWO, Netherlands Organization for Scientific Research. I would like to thank M. Verbruggen and R.T.J. Cappers for unpublished data and C.C. Bakels, L.P. Louwe Kooijmans and L.W.S.W. Amkreutz for useful comments.

References

Bakels, C. 2006. 'Pollen analysis and the reconstruction of the former vegetation', in Louwe Kooijmans, L. P. and Jongste, P. F. B. (eds) *Schipluiden: A Neolithic Settlement on the Dutch North Sea Coast, c. 3500 cal*BC, Analecta Praehistorica Leidensia 37/38 (Leiden), 305–315.

Bakels, C. C. and Van Beurden, L. M. 2001. 'Archeobotanie', in Louwe Kooijmans, L. P. (ed.) *Hardinxveld-Giessendam Polderweg*, RAM 83 (Amersfoort), 325–378.

Bakels, C. C., Van Beurden, L. M. and Vernimmen, T. J. J. 2001. 'Archeobotanie', in Louwe Kooijmans, L. P. (ed.) *Hardinxveld-Giessendam De Bruin*, RAM 88 (Amersfoort), 369–434.

Barker, G. 2006: *The Agricultural Revolution in Prehistory: Why Did Foragers Became Farmers?* (Oxford).

Bastiaens, J., Deforce, K., Klinck, B., Meersschaert, L., Verbruggen, C. and Vrydaghs, L. 2005. 'Palaeobotanical analyses', in Crombé, Ph. (ed.) *The Last Hunter-Gatherer-Fishermen in Sandy Flanders (NW Belgium)* (Ghent), 251–278.

De Hingh, A. E. 2000. *Food Production and Food Procurement in the Bronze Age and Early Iron Age (2000–500 BC)* (Leiden).

Dietsch, M. F. 1996. 'Gathered fruits and cultivated plants at Bercy (Paris), a Neolithic village in a fluvial context', *Vegetation History and Archaeobotany* 5 (1–2), 89–97.

Gehasse, E. F. 1995. *Ecologisch-Archeologisch Onderzoek van het Neolithicum en de Vroege Bronstijd in de Noordoostpolder met de Nadruk op Vindplaats P14*. Upublished PhD Thesis, University of Amsterdam.

Guiran, A. J. and Brinkkemper, O. 2007. *Rotterdam-Randstadrail: Archaeologisch Onderzoek 1 Emplacement Centraal Station*, BOOR rapporten 318 (Rotterdam).

Jones, G. and Rowley-Conwy, P. 2007. 'On the importance of cereal cultivation in the British Neolithic', in Colledge, S. and Conolly, J. (eds) *The Origins and Spread of Domestic Plants in Southwest Asia and Europe* (California), 391–419.

Koot, H. and Van der Have, B. 2001. *Graven in Rijswijk. De Steentijdmensen van Ypenburg* (Rijswijk).

Kroll, H. 2007. 'The plant remains from the Neolithic Funnel Beaker site of Wangels in Holsatia, northern Germany', in Colledge, S. and Conolly, J. (eds) *The Origins and Spread of Domestic Plants in Southwest Asia and Europe* (California), 349–357.

Kubiak-Martens, L. 2006a. 'Botanical remains and plant food subsistence', in Louwe Kooijmans, L. P. and Jongste, P. F. B. (eds.) *Schipluiden: A Neolithic Settlement on the Dutch North Sea Coast, c. 3500 cal*BC, Analecta Praehistorica Leidensia 37/38 (Leiden), 317–338.

Kubiak-Martens, L. 2006b. 'Roots, tubers and processed plant food in the local diet', in Louwe Kooijmans, L. P. and Jongste, P. F. B. (eds) *Schipluiden: A Neolithic Settlement on the Dutch North Sea Coast, c. 3500 cal*BC, Analecta Praehistorica Leidensia 37/38 (Leiden), 339–352.

Larsson, L. 1990. 'The Mesolithic of southern Scandinavia', *Journal of World Prehistory* 4 (3), 257–309.

Louwe Kooijmans, L. P. and Jongste, P. F. B. 2006. *Schipluiden: A Neolithic Settlement on the Dutch North Sea Coast, c. 3500 cal*BC, Analecta Praehistorica Leidensia 37/38 (Leiden).

Louwe Kooijmans, L. P. 2007: 'The gradual transition to farming in the Lower Rhine Basin', in Whittle, A. and Cummings, V. (eds) *Going Over: The Mesolithic-Neolithic Transition in North-West Europe* (Oxford), 287–309.

Luijten, H. 1987. *Palaeobotanische Analyse van enkele Vroeg-Neolithische Afvallagen van Zuiderbuurt I (Noordoostpolder)*, Unpublished report IPP, University of Amsterdam (Amsterdam).

Out, W. A. 2008. 'Neolithisation at the site Brandwijk-Kerkhof, the Netherlands: natural vegetation, human impact and plant food subsistence', *Vegetation History and Archaeobotany* 17 (1), 25–39.

Out, W. A. in press. 'Growing habits? Delayed introduction of crop cultivation at marginal Neolithic wetland sites', *Vegetation History and Archaeobotany*, DOI: 10.1007/s00334-008-0152-Z.

Pals, J. 1984. 'Plant remains from Aartswoud, a Neolithic settlement in the coastal area', in Van Zeist, W. and Casparie, W. A. (eds) *Plants and Ancient Man: Studies in Palaeoethnobotany* (Rotterdam), 313–321.

Perry, D. 1999. 'Vegetative tissues from Mesolithic sites in the Northern Netherlands', *Current Anthropology* **40** (2), 231–237.

Perry, D. 2002. 'Preliminary results of an archaeobotanical analysis of Mesolithic sites in the Veenkoloniën, Province of Groningen, the Netherlands', in Mason, S. L. R. and Hather, J. G. (eds) *Hunter-Gatherer Archaeobotany: Perspectives from the Northern Temperate Zone* (London), 108–116.

Peters, F. J. C. and Peeters, J. H. M. 2001. *De Opgraving van de Mesolithische en Neolithische Vindplaats Urk-E4 (Domineesweg, gemeente Urk)*, RAM 93 (Amersfoort).

Raemaekers, D. C. M. 1999. *The Articulation of a 'New Neolithic': The Meaning of the Swifterbant Culture for the Process of Neolithisation in the Western Part of the North European Plain (4900–3400 BC)* (Leiden).

Raemaekers, D. C. M., Bakels, C. C., Beerenhout, B., Van Gijn, A. L., Hänninen, K., Molenaar, S., Paalman, D., Verbruggen, M. and Vermeeren, C. 1997. 'Wateringen 4: a settlement of the Middle Neolithic Hazendonk 3 Group in the Dutch coastal area', *Analecta Praehistorica Leidensia* **29**, 143–192.

Robinson, M. A. 2000. 'Further considerations of Neolithic charred cereals, fruits and nuts', in Fairbairn, A. S. (ed.) *Plants in Neolithic Britain and Beyond* (Oxford), 85–90.

Robinson, D. E. 2007. 'Exploitation of plant resources in the Mesolithic and Neolithic of southern Scandinavia: from gathering to harvesting', in Colledge, S. and Conolly, J. (eds) *The Origins and Spread of Domestic Plants in Southwest Asia and Europe* (California), 359–374.

Rowley-Conwy, P. 2004. 'How the west was lost: a reconsideration of cultural origins in Britain, Ireland and Southern Scandinavia', *Current Anthropology* **45**, 83–99.

Stevens, C. J. 2007. 'Reconsidering the evidence: towards an understanding of the social contexts of subsistence production in Neolithic Britain', in Colledge, S. and Conolly, J. (eds) *The Origins and Spread of Domestic Plants in Southwest Asia and Europe* (California), 375–389.

Thomas, J. 1999. *Understanding the Neolithic* (London).

Van Gijn, A. L. and Houkes, R. 2006. 'Stone, procurement and use', in Louwe Kooijmans, L. P. and Jongste, P. F. B. (eds) *Schipluiden: A Neolithic Settlement on the Dutch North Sea Coast, c. 3500 cal BC*, Analecta Praehistorica Leidensia 37/38 (Leiden), 167–193.

Van Gijn, A. L., Louwe Kooijmans, L. P. and Zandstra, J. G. 2001. 'Natuursteen', in Louwe Kooijmans, L. P. (ed.) *Hardinxveld-Giessendam Polderweg*, RAM 83 (Amersfoort), 163–179.

Van Haaster, H. 2001. *Archeobotanisch Onderzoek naar de Neolithische Bewoning op de Vindplaats Rijswijk-Ypenburg*, Biaxiaal 118 (Zaandam).

Van der Woude, J. D. 1983. *Holocene Paleoenvironmental Evolution of a Perimarine Fluviatile Area*, Analecta Praehistorica Leidensia 16 (Leiden).

Van Zeist, W. and Palfenier-Vegter, R. M. 1981. 'Seeds and fruits from the Swifterbant S3 site', *Palaeohistoria* **23**, 105–168.

Visser, D., Whitton, C., Brinkkemper, O. and Hogestijn, J. W. H. 2001. 'Archeobotanie: de analyse van botanische macroresten', in Hogestijn, J. W. H. and Peeters, J. H. M. (eds) *De Mesolithische en Vroeg-Neolithische Vindplaats Hoge Vaart-A27 (Flevoland)*, RAM 79 (11) (Amersfoort).

Dinner at the Edge of the World: Why the Greenland Norse Tried to Eat a European Diet in an Unforgiving Landscape

Elizabeth Pierce,
University of Glasgow

Introduction
Scandinavian expansion into the North Atlantic was first recorded in AD 793 when the priory of Lindisfarne, off the coast of present-day Northumbria, was raided by Vikings (Graham-Campbell and Batey 1998, 24). Within a few decades the Vikings (Scandinavians) had rounded the coast of Scotland, established control of many of the islands of the Northern and Western Isles, and had founded settlements in Ireland (such as Dublin and Cork) that later became important trade centres. Joined by other Scandinavians as well as Gaelic settlers and slaves, they spread to the Faroe Islands around AD 825, colonizing Iceland nearly half a century later (Jones 1984, 279; Arge 2000, 154; Vésteinsson 2000, 164).

When the Vikings, or 'Norse' (individuals of Scandinavian descent and cultural identity), first settled in Greenland, *ca.* AD 985, they apparently intended to continue the subsistence practices of their homelands; never adapting their foodways or lifestyles despite the increasingly harsh climate and limited resources of Greenland, unlike the Icelanders and Faroese who altered their traditional subsistence methods and took up large-scale fishing. Instead, the Greenlanders expended precious resources to display their European identity and status in ways that were ill-suited to their sub-Arctic landscape. This stubbornness may have been one factor which contributed to the ultimate decline and disappearance of the Greenland Norse.

Settlement and Subsistence in Greenland
The Viking expansion in the North Atlantic is unique because it is the only case of medieval Europeans colonizing largely uninhabited landscapes. In Greenland there were signs of the previous inhabitants, but the landscape appears to have been empty at the time of settlement. At this point Greenland's climate was slightly warmer than today, the growing season was potentially longer and there was less sea ice to impede sailing. The interior was, however, dominated by an ice sheet, rendering the sheltered fjords along the coast the most hospitable areas for colonization. The Norse built their farms in two main areas: the Eastern Settlement, on the western coast near the southern tip of Greenland, and the Western Settlement, a smaller occupation approximately 400–

500 km north of the Eastern Settlement. Rather than villages like those in medieval Europe, the settlements were series of farms spread through some of the western fjords of Greenland. The best farms stood at the heads of fjords and the others filled the inner-fjord areas of the settlements almost completely (McGovern 1980, 249–250). No primary written sources survive to tell us why the Greenlanders chose this settlement pattern but McGovern (1980, 249) argues that their decisions were based on the subsistence strategies brought from Iceland and that they choose to locate their farms on the best available pasture for cattle, sheep and goats. Proximity to the plentiful supply of marine resources was seemingly less of a priority but the establishment of landing places for incoming trade was important to the Greenland Norse.

Contact with Europe and the other North Atlantic colonies was frequent at first because the Greenland settlers imported from the east goods that they could not manufacture themselves, including necessities such as iron tools and church furnishings (Larson 1917, 142). The colonists submitted to Norwegian (and later Danish) rule and a royal trade monopoly for their imports and exports in the 1260s. Imports came at a high cost to the residents but, early in their settlement, the Greenlanders had resources valuable enough to entice European merchants to make the hazardous journey. Exports included walrus ivory and skin rope, woollen cloth, polar bear skins and the occasional live polar bear, falcons, and narwhal tusks, which in Europe were thought to be unicorn horns (Larson 1917, 142; Jones 1984, 163, 293; Roesdahl 2004, 145).

Despite the importance of outside trade to the Greenlanders, it was not imperative for their survival. Life in Greenland was not difficult prior to the climatic cooling of the fourteenth century. *The King's Mirror*, a thirteenth-century treatise on medieval life in the north, reported 'the pasturage is good and … there are large and fine farms in Greenland' (Larson 1917, 145). Farmers raised cattle, goats and sheep, which they used for meat, wool and especially the milk for butter and cheese (Larson 1917). Pigs, dogs and horses appear in the faunal record, but they did not contribute much to the Norse diet (McGovern 1980, 251; Christensen 1991, 158). The Norse also gathered shellfish and berries, and hunted caribou, seals and other game which could have potentially brought them into contact with the 'native' Thule who arrived in the late thirteenth or early fourteenth centuries (Christensen 1991, 158; Gulløv 2000, 323).

Whilst local food resources were plentiful, the retention of traditional Norse subsistence practices seems to have been important for the Greenland farmers, who apparently attempted to maintain similar subsistence practices to those employed in Iceland. At the élite Western Settlement farm of Sandnes (V51), for example, the eleventh-century domesticate bone assemblage was reminiscent of ninth/tenth-century assemblages from southern Icelandic farms (McGovern 2000, 332). This is interesting given that, by the eleventh century, subsistence strategies in Iceland were themselves changing, possibly due to climatic deterioration: zooarchaeological assemblages from farms in north-eastern and eastern Iceland suggest a substantial decline in cattle remains (from over 40 per cent to just a few per cent) with pigs becoming almost entirely absent (McGovern 2000).

In Greenland, wealthier farms appeared to have continued traditional subsistence more successfully than smaller farms, whose occupants would have been more concerned about basic survival. In particular, high-status sites appear to be associated with cattle and beef seems to have been a high-status food: isotopic analysis of a bishop's skeleton from Garðar has suggested that he consumed more beef and cheese than the average Greenlander, probably a reflection of his social position (Arneborg *et al.* 1999, 164). The concept that cattle equalled wealth was common across the North Atlantic and, although cattle were poorly suited to the Greenland's environment, their importance on the island was probably preserved because money and bullion were not used (McGovern 1980, 260). An indication of their status-associations is clear from the fact that richer Greenlandic farms, especially those with ecclesiastical centres, raised and consumed many more cattle than average farms on the island (McGovern 1980, 261). At Sandnes for instance, cattle bone constituted 17 per cent of the midden material, far higher than at the Western Settlement's inland farms (around nine per cent), and the poor coastal farm labelled V48 where cattle comprised just two to five per cent of the midden assemblage (McGovern 1980, 252). Inland farms compensated for their lack of cattle by raising a higher proportion (20–33 per cent) of sheep and goats, although caprines were also well represented at Sandnes where their representation increased slightly from the eleventh to the fourteenth centuries (McGovern 2000, 333).

Concentration on livestock grazing gradually eroded pastures but because livestock represented status as well as an important source of food, Norse farmers persistently overgrazed, degrading what was already a delicate landscape (McGovern *et al.* 1988, 231). Problems were perhaps greatest in the Western Settlement where, being *ca.* 500 km north of the Eastern Settlement, the growing season was approximately one month shorter, the vegetation was thinner, and the snow line was lower, making it more difficult to grow the fodder necessary to keep livestock alive through the long winters (McGovern 1980, 246; Christensen 1991, 163–164). This may have been one factor causing the abandonment of the Western Settlement before the Eastern Settlement.

Even from the beginning, 'Scandinavian stockraising was clearly near its limits in Greenland' (McGovern 1980, 255). Milk production would have stopped sometime during the winter and, even with the coming of spring, farmers would still have to wait for pastures to regenerate before cattle could be returned to them for grazing. Sheep and goats were more resilient, but an epidemic amongst the livestock or cooler temperatures slowing the growth of grass could quickly prove devastating. A high rate of neonatal cattle and caprine bones show that Norse farmers in Greenland either had trouble producing viable new livestock or needed to kill the neonates so they could feed themselves with the dairy products (McGovern 1980, 255). Many scholars (for instance Christensen 1991, 158) have argued that grain production was also problematic in Greenland, unlike Iceland and the other North Atlantic settlements, because of the climate – it is too far north and too cold (Vésteinsson 2000, 164). One written source notes there were attempts to grow grain in Greenland by some of the wealthiest men there (Larson

1917, 142). However, their experiments failed and grain had to be imported, probably from Britain or Norway. *The King's Mirror* notes that, 'The great majority do not know what bread is, having never seen it' (Larson 1917, 142). This may be an exaggeration but grain would rarely have been eaten by humans. Kevin Edwards of the University of Aberdeen notes that archaeologists who have recently worked in Greenland have seen barley being grown and harvested before ripening as feed for livestock (14.4.2007, 'Recent Developments in North Atlantic Studies' conference, Aberdeen). Perhaps the Norse also did this on occasion to supplement winter fodder, but a scarcity of storable grain for humans meant the Greenlanders would have to depend upon stored meat and dairy products to buffer them against shortages during winter (McGovern 1980, 257). The Norse in Greenland were vulnerable (Buckland *et al.* 1996, 94; McGovern 2000, 334) but they continued to rely on cattle and sheep instead of abandoning domestic livestock for a diet of strictly local origin.

Poorer farms appear to have made more use of locally-available resources. At V48, for instance, seal bones comprised 66–77 per cent of the assemblage, whereas the Sandnes assemblages contained just 18 per cent seal remains (McGovern 1980, 252). Seals seemed to take the place of fish in the Norse diet but on the wealthier sites, that had the means to produce surpluses, the use of seals held steady or even decreased when compared to domestic taxa and caribou in the eleventh to fourteenth centuries. At the same period in Iceland, fish made up more than half of the assemblages while the utilization of seals was very small (McGovern 2000, 333). Of the seals found in middens in Greenland, the most common species are the harp seal (*Phoca groenlandica*) and common seal (*Phoca vitulina*), which were utilized more heavily here than other parts of the North Atlantic (McGovern 1980, 251–252; 2000, 332). While these seal species can live near the settlement areas, they are usually located closer to the ocean (McGovern 1980, 253). Rather than taking animals by boats and harpoons, the Norse hunters apparently used nets and clubs to gather seals; analysis of faunal remains show that most common seals were taken from their pupping grounds, when the animals would have been easy targets (Buckland *et al.* 1996, 94). One species rarely found in the faunal record is the ringed seal (*Pusa hispida*), which is best hunted with a harpoon at a breathing hole, a method employed by the native Thule (McGovern 1980, 265–266; 2000, 336). Ringed seals would have given the Norse an important food source during the winter, when sources of dairy products dried up and they were reliant on stored food (McGovern 2000, 336). Their decision to shun this food source is interesting.

Fish would also seem to be a logical food source for the Greenland Norse based on their proximity to water and utilization of seals. Oddly, evidence for fish in the diet is lacking: fish bones and fishing paraphernalia are rarely found on Norse sites (Buckland *et al.* 1996, 94). Isotope analysis of 27 human bones from Norse Greenland did find that the marine portion of the diet increased over time, but based on midden remains this probably came from seals (Arneborg *et al.* 1999, 160, 165). At the Farm Beneath the Sand, 166 fragments of fish bone were found, by far the largest number of any Norse site in Greenland (Enghoff 2003, 47). Since most of these fragments were recovered by sieving, it could be argued that the majority of fishbone evidence was simply missed in earlier excavations, but this seems unlikely given the general lack of fishing gear.

McGovern (1980, 250) points out that, unlike the rest of their North Atlantic counterparts, the Greenland Norse were dependent upon animal husbandry and hunting without reliable outside connections to supplement their subsistence. Because the Greenland Norse continued to integrate European trends such as wool liripipe hoods and contemporary church architecture into their society, it is surprising they did not follow the medieval Scandinavian trend toward a fishing-based subsistence strategy rather than continuing to rely so much on domestic livestock. Ignoring such a bountiful resource just outside their doors seems strange, but it may be due partly to status and old habits. James Barrett *et al.* (2001, 152) suggest that, during the Viking Period in the Northern Isles of Scotland, fish may have been considered inferior in status to other meat. While fish in the diet and as a trade-good became important during the Middle Ages all the way from Iceland to northern Norway, Greenland never adopted this tradition (Barrett *et al.* 2001; McGovern 2000, 332–333). A lack of ships and poor sea-ice conditions probably left Greenlanders unable to transport dried fish to the medieval markets of Europe, but importation of fish is also unlikely as it was a bulky but lightweight and low-cost commodity for which merchants would not have risked the hazardous journey. The absence of a large-scale fishing industry in Greenland is understandable given the circumstances, but lack of fish for everyday eating is not. In the same way that cattle continued to represent wealth in Greenland, perhaps fish was still perceived as a low-status food and was never adopted into the diet as a staple. Since fish was apparently overlooked but high-status cattle production and traditional sheep and goat production continued, status and cultural identity appear to have been important to the Greenlanders.

The Church

The Church influenced people's lives in the Middle Ages, including diet. One issue was fast days: nearly every major element of the Greenland Norse diet was banned then. According to the Icelandic law-book *Grágás*, banned foods in medieval Iceland included dairy products, meat from all domestic, marine and land mammals, and talon-footed birds, but fish and web-footed birds were allowed (Gad 1970, 84; Dennis *et al.* 1980, 48). Eating meat was allowed only if the alternative was starvation, and offenders were required to atone for such actions (Dennis *et al.* 1980, 48). The new environment in Greenland even led the Church to debate whether whales and walrus were fish, an acceptable food: they decided that whales were fish, but walrus were not (Larson 1917, 140–141). If these rules applied to Greenland, where fish did not comprise a large part of the diet, did the inhabitants go hungry on fast days, or did they simply ignore the Church's rules?

The Greenlanders seemed eager to demonstrate their Christian devotion, expending large amounts of resources to import church bells and stained glass, and building large stone churches based on contemporary plans from Europe (McGovern 1980, 264; Keller 1991, 126). Outside witnesses verified that proper Church protocol was followed for events such as the 1408 wedding at Hvalsey church (Jones 1984: 310; Keller 1991: 127; Arneborg 2000, 316). Throughout the centuries the Greenlanders apparently took Church doctrine seriously enough to follow proper protocols and stay in good standing with the main body of the Church. But many of the farms lay at a distance from ecclesiastical centres and bishops were often absent. Because of the lack of written sources, it is not clear whether they felt compelled to practice the same religious devotion at home as in their churches. Unless special concessions were made for them, one would guess the Greenlanders did not follow fasting rules given the make-up their middens.

Decline and Disappearance

The disappearance of the Greenland Norse is perhaps the most intriguing mystery in North Atlantic archaeology. The fall of the settlements began in the mid-fourteenth century with the abandonment of the Western Settlement, just as the climate was becoming much cooler. The last recorded contact with Greenland was in 1409, and the remaining settlers disappeared sometime between the mid-fifteenth and early-sixteenth century. A range of factors contributed to their disappearance, but no one knows what happened to the last Norse in Greenland (for a summary of current theories, see Lynnerup 1998, 120–128).

Their material culture and lifestyle did not change drastically even as their society collapsed, perhaps in order to display their continuing affiliation with Christianity and Europe. Because of a lack of available imports and only occasional contact with Europe, the Greenlanders used what they could to create modern European fashions out of available materials, such as whalebone belt buckles and necklaces woven from human hair (Arneborg 2000, 314; Østergård 2004, 108). Preserved textiles from the cemetery at Herjolfsnes show that the Norse were constructing fashionable clothing from European patterns out of locally woven wool fabric (Nordtorp-Madson 2000, 55–58).

Their diet likewise retained its connection to the homeland. In the face of a declining society and cooling temperatures, the Norse responded by intensifying their subsistence strategies rather than adapting to new conditions (McGovern 1980, 270). There is no evidence that they turned to harpoon-hunting or fishing even then. The human population was declining and their ability to raise livestock was strained by erosion and less available fodder. There is no sign that they moved to neighbouring fjords or congregated near fjord entrances: McGovern (1980) argues that large ceremonial architecture and a settlement strategy covering most of the inner fjord areas prevented them from seeking new settlement sites from which they could adapt their subsistence strategies to things such as new seal migratory patterns. But a few buildings and a settlement tradition should not be enough to keep a hungry community rooted in place. Unless compelling new evidence can be found to explain this lack of adjustment, it would appear that the Greenlanders were making a cultural decision rather than an economic one.

Conclusions

That the later Greenlanders seemed to continue an old subsistence strategy from home when it was not the most economic means of survival suggests theirs was a society under pressure. Groups tend to display their identifying characteristics most publicly when they feel their survival as a group is threatened in order to define the boundaries between themselves and other groups (Fenton 2003, 6–7, 114), or perhaps in this case, to prove their continued association with Christian Europe. They imported the 'ideal farmyard' and continued to regard cattle as high-status indicators, foregoing much fishing or native hunting techniques and clothing. The cultural changes needed in order for them to continue surviving in Greenland may have been too much to ask.

Throughout the centuries, the Greenland Norse continued to use domestic livestock to add meat and dairy products to their diet even when it was not a suitable strategy for their environment. Grain and most fresh fruits and vegetables would have been nearly absent. Although seals became one of their main foods, the Norse Greenlanders never followed the trend of other parts of the North Atlantic in making fish a sizable part of their diet.

Based on their behavior in subsistence and material culture, it appears diet was a cultural choice rather than an economic one. McGovern (2000, 339) writes: 'When faced with multiple challenges to the basic environmental and social framework of their economy and society, the Norse Greenlanders chose to avoid innovation, to emphasize and elaborate their traditions, and ultimately to die rather than abandon what they must have seen as core values.' Whatever their fate, it is clear that they chose not to adapt their lifestyle fully to the Arctic conditions around them. If their goal was keeping their European roots alive then they succeeded, but their success came at a very high price.

Acknowledgements

This work has been carried out with support from the Sue Green Bursary at the University of Glasgow. The author also would like to thank Erin McGuire, Adrian Maldonado and especially Dr Colleen Batey for their assistance while this paper was written.

References

Arge, S. 2000. 'Vikings in the Faeroe Islands', in W. Fitzhugh and Ward, E. (eds) *Vikings: The North Atlantic Saga* (London), 154–163.

Arneborg, J. 2000. 'Greenland and Europe', in W. Fitzhugh and Ward, E. (eds) *Vikings: The North Atlantic Saga* (London), 304–317.

Arneborg, J., Heinemeier, J., Lynnerup, N., Nielsen, H., Rud, N. and Sveinbjörnsdóttir, Á. 1999. 'Change of diet of the Greenland Vikings determined from stable isotope analysis and 14c dating of their bones', *Radiocarbon* **41** (2), 157–168.

Barrett, J., Beukens, R. and Nicholson, R. 2001. 'Diet and ethnicity during the Viking colonization of northern Scotland: evidence from fish bones and stable carbon isotopes', *Antiquity* **75** (287), 145–154.

Buckland, P., Amorosi, T., Barlow, L., Dugmore, A., Mayewski, P., McGovern, T., Ogilvie, A., Sadler, J. and Skidmore, P. 1996. 'Bioarchaeological and climatological evidence for the fate of Norse farmers in medieval Greenland', *Antiquity* **70**, 88–96.

Christensen, K. M. B. 1991. 'Aspects of the Norse economy in the Western Settlement in Greenland', *Acta Archaeologica* **61**, 158–165.

Dennis, A., Foote, P. and Perkins, R. (trans.) 1980. *Laws of Early Iceland: Grágás* (Winnipeg).

Enghoff, I. 2003. *Hunting, Fishing and Animal Husbandry at The Farm Beneath The Sand, Western Greenland: An Archaeological Analysis of a Norse Farm in the Western Settlement* (Copenhagen).

Fenton, S. 2003. *Ethnicity* (Cambridge).

Gad, F. 1970. *The History of Greenland*, Vol. I (London).

Graham-Campbell, J. and Batey, C. 1998. *Vikings in Scotland: An Archaeological Survey* (Edinburgh).

Gulløv, H. 2000. 'Natives and Norse in Greenland', in Fitzhugh, W. and Ward, E. (eds) *Vikings: The North Atlantic Saga* (London), 318–326.

Jones, G. 1984. *A History of the Vikings*, 2nd edition (Oxford).

Keller, C. 1991. 'Vikings in the West Atlantic: a model of Norse Greenlandic medieval society'. *Acta Archaeologica* **61**, 126–140.

Larson, L. (trans.) 1917. *The King's Mirror – Speculum Regale* (New York).

Lynnerup, N. 1998. *The Greenland Norse: A Biological-anthropological Study*. Meddelelser om Grønland, Man and Society 24 (Copenhagen).

McGovern, T. 1980: 'Cows, harp seals, and churchbells: adaptation and extinction in Norse Greenland', *Human Ecology* **8** (3), 245–275.

McGovern, T. 2000: 'The demise of Norse Greenland', in Fitzhugh, W. and Ward, E. (eds) *Vikings: The North Atlantic Saga* (London), 327–339.

McGovern, T., Bigelow, G., Amorosi, T. and Russell, D. 1988. 'Northern islands, human error, and environmental degradation: a view of social and ecological change in the medieval North Atlantic'. *Human Ecology* **16** (3), 225–270.

Nordtorp-Madson, M. 2000. 'The cultural identity of the late Greenland Norse', in Appelt, M., Berglund, J. and Gulløv, H. (eds) *Identities and Cultural Contacts in the Arctic* (Copenhagen), 55–60.

Roesdahl, E. 2004. 'Walrus ivory and other northern luxuries: their importance for Norse voyages and settlements in Greenland and America', in Lewis-Simpson S. (ed.) *Vinland Revisited* (St. John's, NL), 145–152.

Vésteinsson, O. 2000. 'The archaeology of *landnám*: early settlement in Iceland', in Fitzhugh W. and Ward, E. (eds), *Vikings: The North Atlantic Saga* (London), 164–174.

Østergård, E. 2004. *Woven into the Earth* (Gylling).

Living and Eating in Viking-Age Towns and their Hinterlands

*Kristopher Poole,
University of Nottingham*

Introduction

Out of the wide range of social and economic developments that took place within Viking-Age England, the explosion of towns is perhaps one of the most dramatic, and most significant. This urban growth was such that, by the time of the Norman Conquest, there were more than 100 places with some claim to be regarded as towns (Richards 2004, 78). As substantial centres of population and, variably, of administration, religion, trade and craft working, they would have not only had a substantial impact on the surrounding countryside, but also on the lifestyles of people moving into them. Despite this, previous studies have largely focused on economic aspects of town development (e.g. Hodges 1982), with a tendency to 'undertake analysis using general economic models rather than contextually-based interpretations' (O'Connor 2002, 4). This paper aims to paint a more rounded picture of life within urban and rural contexts, paying attention to both economic and social concerns, considering the nature of rural-urban interactions, and exploring the possibility that regional, even culture-based, variations existed. To achieve this, animal bone data synthesized from 11 rural and 36 urban assemblages dating to the Mid-Saxon (*ca.* AD 650–850) and Viking-Age (*ca.* AD 850–1066) periods are considered. In order to highlight Viking influence, or lack thereof, the data are examined on a geographical basis, assemblages divided into two groups according to whether they derive from sites within (northern/eastern England) or outside (southern/western England) the area of the Danelaw. By so doing, I hope to demonstrate the impact of Scandinavian settlement on the economy and, more importantly, highlight the potential of zooarchaeological evidence to inform about social structures and ideologies in the 'Viking Age'.

Viking Traditions and the Economy of England

In Scandinavia, despite much regional variation, it would seem that great emphasis was placed on animal husbandry, with bones of the three main domesticates – cattle, caprines (sheep and goats) and pigs – usually being the most frequently recovered. However, proportions of each species varied across the Viking world. In Denmark and southern Sweden, cattle seem to have been the most frequently kept species, followed by pigs and then caprines (Randsborg 1985, 239), although sheep/goats are generally better represented on rural, compared to urban, sites. At some (mostly urban) sites,

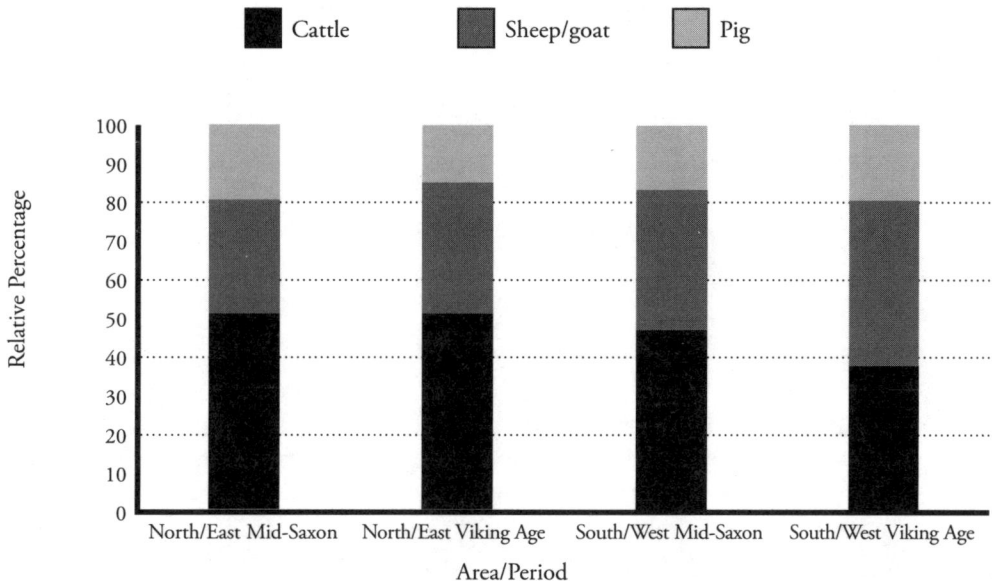

Figure 11.1. Relative frequencies of main domesticates in north/east and south/west England from the Mid-Saxon to Viking-Age periods. Source: Poole (in prep.).

pigs were even the dominant species, as at Birka, Sweden (Wigh 2001) and Kaupang, Norway (Barrett *et al.* 2007). Whilst this may in part be related to environmental conditions, it is notable that cattle were the most frequent species in Iceland, despite the environment being better suited to other forms of subsistence (Vésteinsson 1998). Cattle also seem to have played an important role for Norse settlers in Greenland, even helping play a part in their downfall there (Pierce, this volume).

The apparent importance of cattle in much of the Viking world led O'Connor (1989a) to suggest that the presence of extremely high frequencies of cattle remains recovered from York and Lincoln indicate Viking influence on diet. However, Sykes (2007, 29) has suggested that, although cattle are better represented in Viking-Age assemblages from Danelaw areas than in those from non-Danelaw regions, the variation is more likely due to wider economic change than Viking influence. This suggestion is supported by figure 11.1, which compares the relative frequencies of cattle, sheep/goats and pigs for northern/eastern and southern/western assemblages dating to the Mid-Saxon and Viking-Age periods. The data actually suggest little inter-period change in cattle proportions for northern/eastern England, the only discernable shift being a four per cent increase in caprines at the expense of pigs. In contrast, for southern/western England, there is a ten per cent rise in sheep/goats, compensated by a decline in cattle, between the Mid-Saxon and Viking-Age periods. At this very general level then, the Scandinavian settlers seem to have had little impact on the frequencies of animals kept in this country.

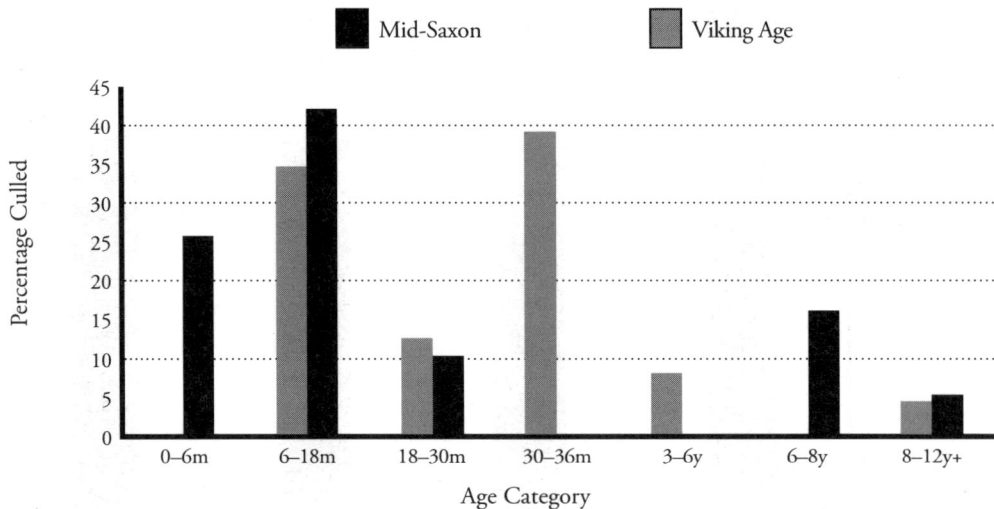

Figure 11.2. Relative frequencies of cattle culled on Mid-Saxon and Viking-Age rural sites in norther/eastern England, by age category. Source: Poole (in prep.).

This could be partly explained by the fact that, in contrast to Greenland and Iceland, the first Scandinavian settlers in England were faced with long-established agricultural regimes and an already intensively-exploited landscape. No doubt the Viking presence caused considerable disruption to farming regimes in some areas but it is likely that, as Hadley (2006, 85) has suggested, the settlers frequently occupied and exploited pre-existing estates. In these cases, they may have chosen to maintain the farming strategies of earlier occupants.

Possible changes in husbandry regimes are very difficult to investigate due to the severe dearth of published reports from rural sites. Although some animals could have been raised in towns (see below), the data from urban sites may reflect marketing choices rather than the economy in the hinterland (O'Connor 1989b, 21). For example, although ageing data from Kaupang, Dorestad and York have been suggested to indicate a focus on beef consumption (Barrett *et al.* 2007, 306), these bones only represent animals being brought in specifically for meat; dairy products such as cheese and butter could have been imported into towns from their hinterlands. Dairy products seem to have played an important role in much of Scandinavian diet (Simpson 1967, 60). In Iceland, for example, the need for quality fodder to produce milk has even been suggested to have determined the initial settlement structure (Vésteinsson 1998). If animals were being kept for dairy purposes, one would expect to find a reasonable proportion of cattle younger than six months, and at least a small number of old cattle with heavily worn teeth; milch cows generally being kept to

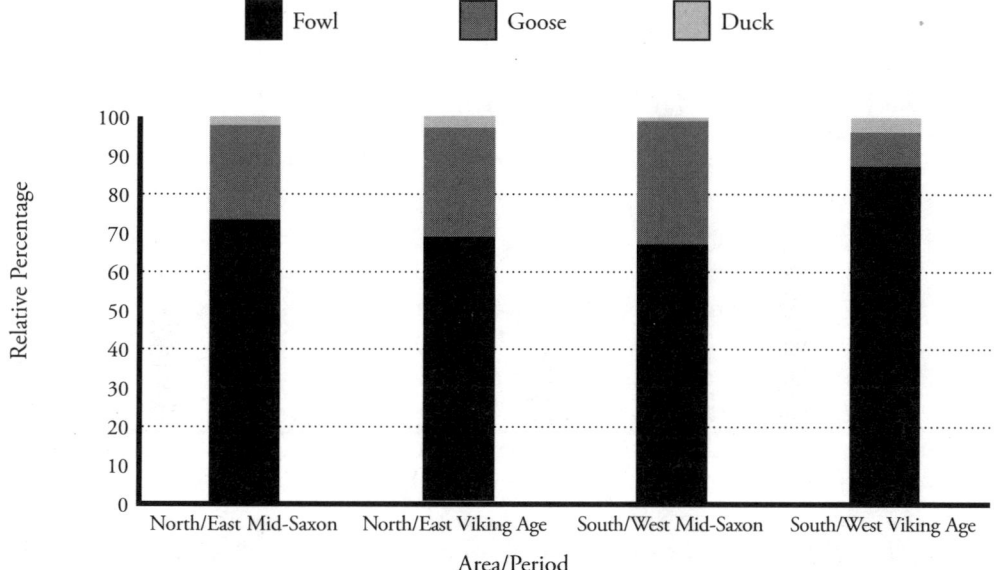

Figure 11.3. Relative frequencies of domestic birds in north/east and south/west England from Mid-Saxon to Viking-Age periods. Source: Poole (in prep.).

an older age than breeding stock. A comparison of ageing data from the very small amount available for northern/eastern England rural sites (Fig. 11.2) could feasibly suggest a shift coinciding with the Viking Age. Unfortunately, it will not be possible to confirm that the shift reflects Viking influence until further data from southern and western sites become available.

Town and Country

So far this paper has dealt with overall trends within the country, but will now focus specifically on urban sites. We must be aware that the division between town and country in the past was not as marked as it is today, where the idea that cities are the exclusive domain of humans is widespread and there are clear ideas about the types of animals suitable and unsuitable for urban environments (Philo 1995; Wolch 2002). However, although Viking-Age towns varied widely in size and population, they represented permanent human settlements where a significant proportion of the population was involved in non-agricultural occupations. This potential difference between town and countryside is important because a person's social position (and occupation) would have affected the types of interactions that they had with animals, and in turn their and others' views of the world (Löfgren 1985). Animals can be encountered by humans in many forms – alive, dead, body parts, raw materials, or art

– and the type of interaction would in turn determine attitudes and responses towards them (for example, Pluskowski 2004).

The move away from full-time agricultural production and towards full-time craft production would, therefore, have been significant, as people began engaging with animals not so much as living creatures, but more often as body-parts (meals, waste), raw materials, and objects. This would, of course, be truer for domestic food species than those animals generally not eaten in this period, both domestic (dogs, cats) and wild (mice, rats, corvids). Increasing craft specialization in the Viking Age, evident in, for example, tenth-century street names in Winchester (such as Tanner Street and Fleshmonger Street) and York (Biddle 1976, 131) must have increased the distance between some humans and animals. To what extent was food being produced within towns? In both north/east and south/west England, cattle, sheep/goats and pigs make up around 93 per cent of the total mammal and bird assemblage. Of the three taxa, cattle are better represented on Viking-Age urban sites, compared to rural sites in both areas. Body-part patterns from towns suggest that the main domesticates were driven in on the hoof. It is known that cattle are easier to drive than sheep/goats or pigs, but they also provide much more meat than a small rural community could have consumed in a short time. Such patterns are also evident at the Scandinavian town of Birka (Wigh 2001). That close urban-rural relationships did exist in England is demonstrated by Alan Vince's (1994) study of tenth- and eleventh-century pottery distributions, which indicates a large amount of traffic between towns and from towns into the countryside.

The extent to which a town depended on food coming in from the surrounding area, and the amount it supplied for itself would have varied depending on size. In Winchester, pressure on space was so intense by the first half of the tenth century that extra-mural suburbs developed (Biddle 1976, 134), in contrast to the byres and agricultural activity evident inside Gloucester's walls (Astill 2000, 36). Relative absence of neonatal and very young animals at some Mid-Saxon urban sites has led some researchers to suggest that animal breeding did not occur within these, or later, towns (for instance Bourdillon 1994, 122). However, lack of evidence for breeding in one area of a town does not mean that it did not occur elsewhere within it (Albarella 2005, 143). The presence of small numbers of mandibles from animals under six months suggests that at least some breeding may have occurred in and around the immediate vicinity of the towns.

Pigs were probably the most common domestic mammal kept in towns, as they can be fed on scraps and do not require the same amount of space as cattle and caprines. High numbers of neonatal pig bones at York suggest that households occasionally obtained a pregnant sow from rural communities, or that pigs were being bred in towns (O'Connor 1989b, 17). Domestic birds could also have contributed a significant proportion to the diet, in the form of both eggs and meat. Chickens were probably the most frequently kept (Fig. 11.3), although geese provide more meat than chickens, and are also a useful source of feathers. It is interesting that geese are retained in northern and eastern towns longer than elsewhere in the country. Grant (1988, 163) suggests the popularity of goose keeping is linked to local environment, with the fenlands of East Anglia and low-lying areas of Lincolnshire providing the kinds of habitat that geese prefer. It is possible, therefore, that this reflects the development of specialized goose breeding in these areas. Due to insufficient data for Scandinavia, it is not currently possible to determine the extent to which Viking influence could also have played a part.

It is clear that the greatest part of the urban dwellers' diet derived from domestic sources supplied from the rural hinterland. This was probably also the case with much of the wild component. In northern/eastern towns, wild species make up only 0.7 per cent of the remains, and only one per cent within south/west towns. Wild species were in fact not regularly consumed at any social level during the Viking Age, but are better represented than in the preceding period, particularly on élite and ecclesiastical sites (Sykes 2005, 86–87). Most of the red deer and roe deer remains from urban sites are antler, often shed, and are not good evidence for venison consumption. One wild resource that town dwellers could have mostly obtained themselves was fish. For most of the Viking Age, the vast majority of fish consumed were freshwater and/or estuarine species (Barrett et al. 2004), which could have been caught from rivers in and around towns. However, around AD 1000, there seems to have been a major shift towards marine species (Barrett et al., 2004), which would have been brought in by outside traders.

Wild birds also provided a very small part of the diet within towns (0.3 per cent of the total bone fragments). As commerce within towns grew, the rise of professional fowlers at least from the late ninth century onwards would have helped vary the urban diet. Fowlers would have used a variety of methods for capturing wild birds, including nets, snares, traps and hawking. The find of a partial goshawk skeleton from Lincoln, as well as goshawk remains from York and Norwich, along with peregrine at Oxford and sparrowhawk at Thetford may all represent birds kept in the town by these fowlers. Alternatively, given the known association between falconry and the social élite during this period, they could have been birds kept by high-status people living in or visiting these towns. In the later Middle Ages, peregrine falcons were used by people of the highest status, whereas sparrowhawks and goshawks could also be used by lower nobility and wealthy commoners (Albarella and Thomas 2002, 25), but whether this hierarchy of birds applied in Viking-Age England is unknown.

The bias of these finds towards towns in the north and east of England is interesting. Hawking was certainly carried out in England before the arrival of the Vikings, but it is possible that Scandinavian influence gave added impetus to its popularity; foreign hawks apparently being particularly prized. The earliest explicit reference to hawking birds being imported to England from Scandinavia is in Domesday Book, which states that the county of Worcester owed the king £10 or a Norway hawk (Oggins 2004, 46), probably a gyrfalcon (Hagen 1995, 146). However, a possible earlier reference is found in King Ethelbert of Kent's letter to St Boniface in Germany (dated ca. AD 748–755) that asks Boniface to send two trained falcons for hunting, the likes of which, according to Ethelbert, are rare in Kent (Oggins 2004, 38). Although the identity of these birds is not given, Dobney and Jacques (2002, 15) suggest that they were 'almost certainly gyrfalcons'. If true, this is interesting, given that these birds live in areas of tundra and mountains, and so were probably long extinct in the British Isles. The nearest sources would therefore have been Scandinavia (Coy, forthcoming). It is possible that Boniface was being asked to act as an intermediary between Ethelbert and Scandinavian traders, although no gyrfalcon remains have yet been identified from Viking-Age deposits in England.

In general, people of high status are almost zooarchaeologically invisible in towns because most animal bone assemblages from urban sites originate from a mixture of different activities and only rarely represent the refuse from a specific family, house or even event. There are, however, some exceptions; Bond and O'Connor (1999), for example, linked variation in bone assemblages from medieval York to known function and status of different areas of the town. The recovery of a pheasant bone from Viking-Age Lincoln (Dobney *et al.* 1996) and of peacock remains from Viking-Age Thetford (Jones 1984) are probably rare direct zooarchaeological evidence of a high-status presence in towns. Although first introduced to Britain during the Roman period, breeding populations of both pheasant and peafowl were probably not established until the later Middle Ages, and so their representation here suggests they were deliberately imported as exotica (Poole, forthcoming). The fact that both examples are from north/east towns may be significant, given the evidence for Viking trade links with the eastern Mediterranean, and the peacock remains and feathers found in the late ninth century Viking ship burial at Gokstad (Brøndsted 1940).

Overall, there is little clear evidence for Viking settlers impacting on diet within England following the settlements, but some of the zooarchaeological data does hint at the presence of Scandinavian settlers at some sites. In England from the eighth century onwards, horse flesh was considered by the Christian Church to be a taboo food (Meens 2002, 4–11). However, horse bones with butchery marks are occasionally found, and it is interesting that eight of the 11 Late Saxon sites with such evidence are within the area of the Danelaw (Poole in prep.): at the urban sites of Norwich, Thetford and York, as well as from the rural site of Sedgeford, Norfolk and the high-status site of Flixborough, Lincolnshire. Butchered horse remains were also recovered from Viking-Age layers at Fishamble Street, Dublin, where three out of 25 disarticulated bones had cut or chop marks, and many other bones had been broken for marrow extraction (McCormick and Murray 2007, 231). In northern Germany and Denmark, the horse was primarily kept for meat and as a status symbol for riding right up until the first millennium AD (Randsborg 1985, 237). The horse also played an important role in Scandinavian society, being used in sacrifice and for horse fights, and the consumption of horse flesh and the slaughter of horses for funerals were also important parts of fertility cults (Sikora 2003–2004, 87). Given this significance, it is possible, although by no means certain, that these finds are evidence of pagan Scandinavian settlers living at these sites.

Conclusion

The Scandinavian settlement of England seems to have had little impact on species proportions overall, although ageing data from rural sites does suggest a potential shift in cattle husbandry regimes. At present, given the lack of published data from rural areas, however, this cannot be attributed to Viking influence. The broad approach taken here also likely masks a much more complex reality, with regional variation. Better-dated assemblages from different areas may help clarify the picture in future. However, if, as has been suggested by Hadley (2006), the settlers often occupied and exploited pre-existing estates, this may explain the lack of evidence for a change in species proportion, with many settlers adapting to the existing system, in order to help them take control. It may also have been the case that the supply of beef was already adequate for their needs; as shown, cattle were already the dominant species in England before their arrival. Indeed, other evidence, such as butchered horse remains, point to the continuation of some dietary practices, at least on occasion.

Towns would have had a real mixture of people from different social levels. However, when considering an urban assemblage, methods of waste disposal, recovery and reporting often mean there is little evidence for social differentiation. In general, the bones recovered during urban excavations will usually only give a general idea of the foods consumed by the town's inhabitants. Moreover, in analysing towns in terms of general economic models, we lose sight of the range of interactions that went on within them. Through considering the evidence at the broadest level, it is hoped that this paper gives some idea of the potential of zooarchaeological remains, and the approach adopted, to help elucidate what it was like to live and work within Viking-Age towns.

References

Albarella, U. 2005. 'Meat production and consumption in town and country', in Giles, K. and Dyer, C. (eds) *Town and Country in the Middle Ages: Contrasts, Contacts and Interconnections, 1100–1500* (Leeds), 131–148.

Albarella, U. and Thomas, R. 2002. 'They dined on crane: bird consumption, wild fowling and status in medieval England', *Acta Zoologica Cracoviensa* **45** (special issue), 23–38.

Astill, G. 2000. 'General survey 600–1300', in Palliser, D. (ed.) *The Cambridge Urban History of Britain. Volume 1: 600–1540* (Cambridge), 27–49.

Barrett, J. H., Hall, A., Johnstone, C., Kenward, H., O'Connor, T. and Ashby, S. 2007. 'Interpreting the plant and animal remains from Viking-age Kaupang', in Skre, D. (ed.) *Kaupang in Skiringssal: Excavation and Surveys at Kaupang and Huseby, 1998–2003. Background and Results* (Aarhus), 283–319.

Barrett, J. H., Locker, A. M. and Roberts, C. M. 2004. "Dark Age Economics' revisited: the English fish bone evidence AD 600–1600', *Antiquity* **78** (301), 618–636.

Biddle, M. 1976. 'Towns', in Wilson, D. M. (ed.) *The Archaeology of Anglo-Saxon England* (London), 99–150.

Bourdillon, J. 1994. 'The animal provisioning of Saxon Southampton', in Rackham, J. (ed.) *Environment and Economy in Anglo-Saxon England* (York), 120–125.

Bond, J. and O'Connor, T. P. 1999. *Bones from Medieval Deposits at 16–22 Coppergate and Other Sites in York* (York).

Brøndsted, J. 1940. *Danmarks Oldtid* (Copenhagen).

Coy, J. forthcoming. 'The Late Saxon and medieval animal bone from the western suburbs', in Serjeantson, D. and Rees, H. (eds), *Food, Craft and Status in Saxon and Medieval Winchester: The Evidence from the Suburbs and City Defences* (Winchester).

Dobney, K. and Jacques, S. D. 2002. 'Avian signatures and status in Anglo-Saxon England', *Acta Zoological Cracoviensia* **45** (special issue), 7–21.

Dobney, K. M., Jacques, S. D. and Irving, B. G. 1996. *Of Butchers and Breeds: Report on Vertebrate Remains from Various Sites in the City of Lincoln* (Lincoln).

Grant, A. 1988. 'The animal resources', in Astill, G. and Grant, A. (eds) *The Countryside of Medieval England* (Oxford), 149–187.

Hadley, D. 2006. *The Vikings in England: Settlement, Society and Culture* (Manchester).

Hagen, A. 1995. *Anglo-Saxon Food and Drink: Processing and Consumption* (Hockwold-cum-Wilton).

Hodges, R. 1982. *Dark Age Economics* (London).

Jones, G. 1984. 'Animal bones', in Rogerson, A. and Dallas, C. (eds) *Excavations in Thetford 1948–59 and 1973–80* (Dereham), 187–192.

Löfgren, O. 1985. 'Our friends in nature: class and animal symbolism', *Ethnos* **50**, 184–213.

McCormick, F. and Murray, E. 2007. *Knowth and the Zooarchaeology of Early Christian Ireland* (Dublin).

Meens, R. 2002. 'Eating animals in the early Middle Ages: classifying the animal world and building group identities', in Creager, A. N. H. and Jordan, W. C. (eds) *The Animal/Human Boundary: Historical Perspectives* (Rochester), 3–28.

O'Connor, T. P. 1989a. *Bones from Anglo-Scandinavian levels at 16–22 Coppergate* (London).

O'Connor, T. P. 1989b. 'What shall we have for dinner? Food remains from urban sites', in Serjeantson, D. and Waldron, T. (eds) *Diet and Crafts in Towns: The Evidence of Animal Remains from the Roman to Post-medieval Periods* (Oxford), 13–23.

O'Connor, T.P. 2002. 'Medieval zooarchaeology: what are we trying to do?', in Pluskowski, A. (ed.) *Archaeological Review from Cambridge* **18**, 3–21.

Oggins, R. 2004. *Kings and Their Hawks: Falconry in Medieval England* (New Haven).

Philo, C. 1995. 'Animals, geography and the city: notes on inclusions and exclusions', *Environment and Planning D: Society and Space* **13** (6), 655–81.

Pluskowski, A. 2004. 'Narwhals or unicorns? Exotic animals as material culture in medieval Europe', *European Journal of Archaeology* **7** (3), 291–313.

Poole, K. forthcoming. 'Bird introductions', in O'Connor, T. P. and Sykes, N. J. (eds) *Invasions and Extinctions: The Social History of British Fauna* (Macclesfield).

Poole, K. in prep. *The Nature of Society in England, c. AD 410–1066*. Unpublished PhD thesis, University of Nottingham.

Randsborg, K. 1985. 'Subsistence and settlement in northern temperate Europe in the first millennium A.D.', in Barker, G. and Gamble, C. (eds) *Beyond Domestication in Prehistoric Europe in the First Millenium A.D.* (London), 233–265.

Richards, J. D. 2004. *Viking Age England* (Stroud).

Sikora, M. 2003–2004. 'Diversity in Viking Age horse burial: A comparative study of Norway, Iceland, Scotland and Ireland', *The Journal of Irish Archaeology* **12–13**, 87–109.

Simpson, J. 1967. *Everyday Life in the Viking Age* (London).

Sykes, N. J. 2005. 'The dynamics of status symbols: wildfowl exploitation in England AD 410–1550', *Archaeological Journal* **161**, 82–105.

Sykes, N. J. 2007. *The Norman Conquest: A Zooarchaeological Pespective* (Oxford).

Vésteinsson, O. 1998. 'Patterns of settlement in Iceland: a study in prehistory', *Saga-Book of Viking Society for Northern Research* **25**, 1–29.

Vince, A. 1994. 'Saxon urban economies: an archaeological perspective' in Rackham, J. (ed.) *Environment and Economy in Anglo-Saxon England* (York), 108–119.

Wigh, B. 2001. *Animal Husbandry in the Viking Age Town of Birka and its Hinterland* (Stockholm).

Wolch, J. 2002. 'Anima urbis', *Progress in Human Geography* **26** (6), 721–742.

Stable Isotope Analysis of Skeletal Remains from Jordan: Environment, Diet and Societies of Past Southern Levant

*Michela Sandias,
University of Reading*

Introduction

Jordan has an exceptional archaeological heritage with sites ranging from the Palaeolithic and some of the earliest known Neolithic settlements, to the Byzantine and Islamic periods, including world famous monuments from Nabataean and Roman times. Jordan is also characterized by a variety of environments of which two extreme examples are the Jordan Valley, situated below sea level, and the Western Highlands (Macumber 2001). Since the Palaeolithic this area has undergone climatic and ecological changes which have coincided with crucial cultural transformations (MacDonald *et al.* 2001). In this setting, dietary reconstruction by carbon and nitrogen stable isotope analysis of human and animal bones from various archaeological sites can inform on the exploitation of resources and on the interaction with different environments in ancient Jordan over an extended period of time. It can also contribute to the knowledge of the culture and socio-economic structure of human groups. This study was conceived in the broad perspective of the multidisciplinary project Water Life and Civilisation (Website 1), which aims to investigate meteorology, hydrology, palaeoenvironments and archaeology in Jordan and to link these themes with prospects of development in the future of this country.

Bone Collagen Stable Isotope Analysis

Stable carbon and nitrogen isotope analysis of bone collagen is a well-established chemical methodology for reconstructing diet directly from human and faunal skeletal remains (Sealy 2001; Ambrose 1993). Stable isotope ratios $^{13}C/^{12}C$ and $^{15}N/^{14}N$ (expressed in ‰, respectively as $\delta^{13}C$ and $\delta^{15}N$ when referred to a standard) measured in human and animal bone collagen reflect the isotopic ratios of the foods, especially of the dietary protein, consumed over an individual's lifetime. Different foods show a range of stable isotope ratios that vary according to the isotopic composition of the environment in which they are produced. Plants are at the base of the foodweb and, dependent on their photosynthetic pathways, they can be distinguished into C_3 and C_4 plants. C_3 plants are typical of winter rainfall, shaded, high latitude and high altitude environments. Most plants used for human consumption are C_3 plants, for example wheat, most fruits, legumes and nuts. C_4 plants are adapted to hot, sunny and dry habitats. They include many tropical grasses but also the important cultural crops of maize, sorghum, millet and sugar cane. Due to their different photosynthetic pathways, C_3 and C_4 plants differ in the $\delta^{13}C$ of their tissues: Smith and Epstein (1971) have shown that C_3 plants have more negative $\delta^{13}C$ values (on average -26‰) than C_4 plants (-12.5 ‰). These differences are transferred to the consumers' body tissue, including their bone collagen. The $\delta^{13}C$ ratios of bone collagen therefore provide a measure of the levels of C_3 and C_4 plants in the diet of herbivores. For humans and other omnivores they may reflect either direct consumption of plants or varying $\delta^{13}C$ ratios of meat or dairy products derived from C_3- or C_4-fed animals (Ambrose 1993).

Ratios of nitrogen stable isotopes are related to the trophic position of an organism in a food web, the $\delta^{15}N$ ratios of body proteins becoming enriched in ^{15}N with each trophic level (Bocherens and Drucker 2003). So, the $\delta^{15}N$ measured in a herbivore is 3–5‰ higher than that of the plants the animal is feeding on. Therefore, in an archaeological study, when nitrogen isotopic ratios from contextual fauna are available, $\delta^{15}N$ ratios of humans can be used to estimate the level of animal products in the diet (Schwarcz and Schoeninger 1991). A negative correlation has been demonstrated between $\delta^{15}N$ and rainfall, $\delta^{15}N$ ratios often being higher in arid environments (Heaton *et al.* 1986, Schwarcz *et al.* 1999). Both $\delta^{13}C$ and $\delta^{15}N$ ratios can be useful to identify consumption of marine or freshwater resources (Schoeninger *et al.* 1983).

Previous Isotope Studies in the Area

To date, few studies of stable isotope analysis have been undertaken for skeletal remains from south-west Asia and northern Africa. Work in Jordan has been carried out by Al-Shorman (2004) who analysed tooth enamel carbonate from the Middle and Late Bronze Age cemetery of Tell Ya'amun. Here isotope data suggested a diet mostly based on C_3 plants. No differences were found between the two Bronze Age phases despite the climate and environmental changes that had occurred. The analysis of carbonate does not allow for the measurement of nitrogen stable isotope ratios and therefore no inferences of levels of plant versus animal protein in the diet could be made. Within the wider context of the Middle East, Richards *et al.* (2003) examined remains from Neolithic Çatalhöyük, Turkey. This study suggested a diverse animal diet which included C_4 plants, especially for the sheep. The human diet included animal and plant proteins, as well as an input of C_4 plants probably due to the consumption of herbivore products. Stable isotope data also demonstrated that, despite the widely-perceived importance of cattle at the site, they did not actually make a significant contribution to human diet (Richards *et al.* 2003).

Up to now, most isotope studies from the region have been carried out on material from Egypt, especially the Nile Valley, which may provide an analogue for environmental conditions in the Jordan Valley (Oleson 2001). The patterns of human diet which have emerged from the studies by Iacumin *et al.* (1996) and Thompson *et al.* (2005) indicate that resources in the Egyptian Nile Valley were dominated by C_3

plant-derived foods. The observed $\delta^{13}C$ and $\delta^{15}N$ ratios were also compatible with the archaeologically-attested importance of freshwater fish consumption, although environmental conditions, aridity in particular, offer an alternative explanation for the high nitrogen isotopic values (Iacumin et al. 1996, Thompson et al. 2005). Further south, in Nubia, the proportion of C_4 plants that directly or indirectly contributed to human diet was greater than in Egypt (Iacumin et al. 1998; Thompson et al. 2007), demonstrating how geography and environmental conditions are reflected in human and animal bone collagen values (van Klinken et al. 2000).

Whilst these studies demonstrate a growing interest in the study of food and consumption practices in the Near and Middle East, there exists great potential for enhancing our understanding of diet in these regions.

A New Study of Food Production and Consumption in Ancient Jordan

Agriculture and rearing of domesticated species have had a very long history in Jordan. Starting from the Bronze Age (ca. 3600 BC to ca. 1200 BC), agricultural productivity was increased by technological innovation, particularly the employment of irrigation. Major cultivated species were cereals and pulses and, among tree crops, olive and vine. Sedentary communities acquired secondary animal products from those involved in livestock management, a practice that also included some form of seasonal movement (Philip 2001).

During the Roman period (63 BC to AD 324), Jordan witnessed an increase in rural settlements and in agricultural activities, a situation perhaps explained by the relative stability brought by the Roman Empire (Freeman 2001). Evidence from Palestine indicates that new rural settlements were preferentially located on hills, with agriculture being practiced in the valleys (Anderson 1998). Organization of domestic buildings shows continuity with the pre-Roman period, attesting that farming was still the basis of household economy (Freeman 2001). In contrast, urban entities such as Pella and Jerash were included in complex road networks and were involved in the trade of agricultural and industrial products (Anderson 1998). With the start of the Byzantine era (AD 324), the region assumed a special role in the empire, the Christian holy places having become the destination of both attention and pilgrimage. This interest entailed economic prosperity that encouraged settlement expansion and increase in population size. Some scholars have argued that a minor change in climate, recorded as slight increase in rainfall and colder temperature, characterized the Byzantine period and might have had a positive influence on both land use and demography; however, evidence for this is still unclear (Patrich 1998). Over-exploitation of the natural environment continued during the Byzantine period when deforestation increased and erosion appeared in certain areas (Watson 2001). Agricultural production was stimulated by urban demand for crops. The range of cultivated products was large: grapes, olives, fruit, nuts and horticultural products are documented, along with cereals (wheat and barley). Evidence for animal husbandry is found in both the countryside

Stable Isotope Analysis of Skeletal Remains from Jordan

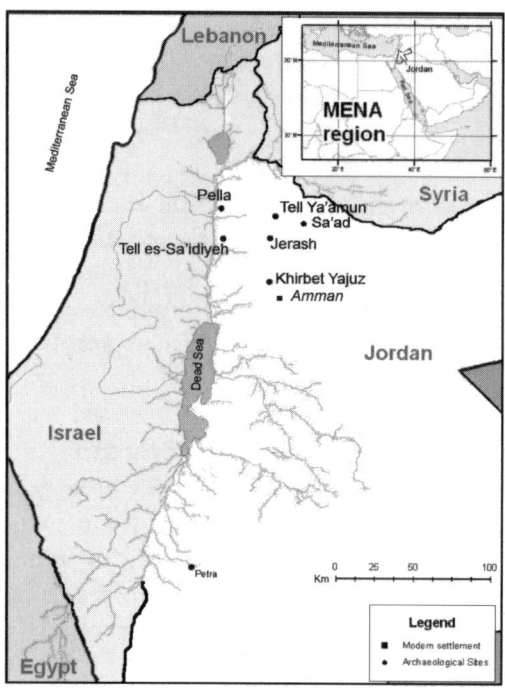

Figure 12.1. Map of Jordan showing the archaeological sites mentioned in the text (modified after the 'Water, Life and Civilisation Annual Report 2006' available at http://www.waterlifecivilisation.org/research/project_publications/annual_reports/year2).

and cities where animals apparently occupied stables at the ground floor of the houses (Watson 2001). Within this picture of general prosperity and stability, disrupting factors such as natural catastrophes, epidemics and Saracen incursions (Patrich 1998) intervened, debilitating the populations and weakening the central administration. The Byzantine era was brought to an end by Muslim conquest in AD 638.

Against this backdrop, the present study will analyse more than 300 archaeological samples from sites in northern Jordan. The sites have been selected on the basis of their type, date and geographical position – because isotopes can help in the identification of ecosystems, sites located in different ecological settings, such as the Western Highlands and the Jordan Valley, have been chosen (see Fig. 12.1). It is hoped that comparison of cities, such as Jerash and Pella, with smaller towns, like Tell Ya'amun, Khirbet Yajuz and Sa'ad, will highlight differences/similarities in rural and urban access to food resources. Issues concerning food production and consumption, both crucial aspects in the cultural and economic structure of a society (Goodman *et al.* 2000), may help to address and evaluate social differentiation, which is expressed also as free or limited access to food resources (Wiessner 1996). The inclusion of multi-period sites, such as Tell Ya'amun, Pella and Tell es-Sa'idiyeh, will offer the opportunity to see whether behaviours relative to food have changed over time and if these changes coincided with transformations in political and economic systems.

The Tell Ya'amun and Khirbet Yajuz Case Studies
Tell Ya'amun and Khirbet Yajuz are both located in the Western Highlands and hence the landscapes that surround them are similar in their altitudinal and climatic characteristics. Evidence from Late Antiquity collected to date suggests that the two sites were also similar in size and economic characterizations.

Tell Ya'amun
Tell Ya'amun was occupied from the Early Bronze Age to the Islamic periods but excavations to date have focused on the Bronze Age, Late Roman and Byzantine occupation layers (El-Najjar *et al.* 2001). Samples of human bone were taken from 15 Late Roman-Byzantine tombs and three Middle Bronze and Late Bronze Age tombs. Amongst the Late Antiquity tombs, the degree of elaboration is very variable, this showing how people, probably from different social ranks, could afford to invest in higher or lower standards of craftsmanship (Rose *et al.* in press).

Khirbet Yajuz
Located a few kilometres north of Amman, the site was described by the first archaeologists as a 'large Romano-Byzantine town' strategically placed along the way connecting Amman (Philadelphia, in antiquity) and Jerash (Suleiman 1996). The main structures excavated at this site are a basilica church and a smaller chapel featuring a hypogean cemetery. Skeletal remains were sampled from the hypogean cemetery where two types of burial have been identified: loculi, which were carved into the rock and possibly used to bury important persons, and constructed graves, thought either to have housed commoners or to have been built in a later phase (Khalil 1998). The uneven distribution of the diverse artefacts and objects of personal adornment recovered from the constructed graves suggests social heterogeneity (Khalil 1998).

Isotopic Values: Results and Discussion
Human stable isotope data from the archaeological sites Tell Ya'amun and Khirbet Yajuz, in northern Jordan, are shown in figure 12.2 (overleaf), where they are compared to the results of studies on human remains from the Nile Valley. Mean values are indicated along with one standard deviation, which represents the variability observed between individuals.

Carbon and nitrogen isotopic values at Tell Ya'amun show little variation between the Bronze Age and the Late Roman-Byzantine populations particularly in the $\delta^{13}C$ values. This similarity in carbon and nitrogen isotopic values over more than 2000 years is striking given that other archaeological and historical evidence suggest that the two periods had different economic systems and resource availability.

The $\delta^{13}C$ values measured in the humans from Tell Ya'amun indicate that, in both periods, human diet was dominated by C_3-derived protein, supporting Al-Shorman's (2004) findings for the Bronze Age period at this site. The $\delta^{15}N$ ratios are compatible

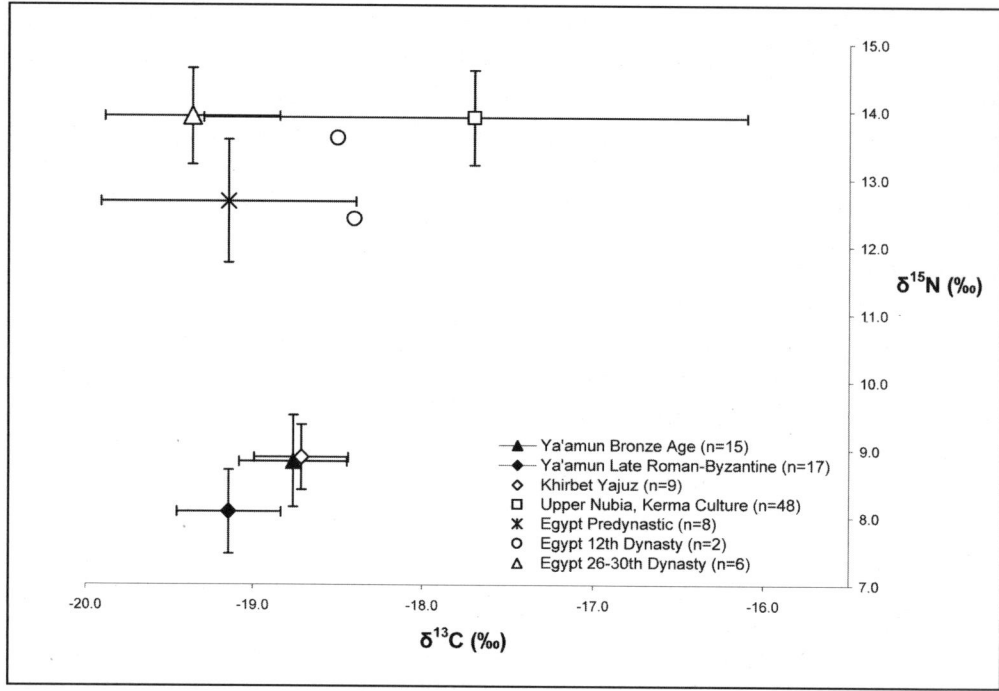

Figure 12.2. Mean $\delta^{13}C$ and $\delta^{15}N$ ratios for the Jordanian sites Tell Ya'amun and Khirbet Yajuz represented with one standard deviation (bars) in comparison with mean ratios from Egypt (after Thompson et al. 2005) and Nubia (after Thompson et al. 2007).

with consumption of a mixture of plant and animal proteins, although the relative contribution of each cannot be determined without background isotopic data from contemporary fauna. Collagen carbon and nitrogen values from the Byzantine site of Khirbet Yajuz plot very close to ratios from Late Roman-Byzantine Tell Ya'amun. Both sites are situated in the Western Highlands region and, according to these preliminary isotopic data, the people buried at these two locations relied on similar resources provided by a predominantly C_3 ecosystem.

Isotopic evidence from Egypt, dating from 5500 BC to 343 BC, testify a C_3-based diet (Thompson *et al.* 2005) very similar to that found for Bronze Age Tell Ya'amun. In contrast, C_4-derived foods certainly contributed to the diet of some individuals from Upper Nubia (Thompson *et al.* 2007). Yet, the less negative $\delta^{13}C$ ratios measured at Tell Ya'amun and Khirbet Yajuz are comparable to values found in human remains from Neolithic Çatalhöyük, for which some intake of C_4-derived foods was suggested, the contextual fauna giving support to this hypothesis (Richards *et al.* 2003). A similar interpretation for the less negative $\delta^{13}C$ values seen at Ya'amun and Yajuz will need isotopic evidence from the fauna to be confirmed.

The $\delta^{15}N$ values of the humans from northern Jordan are unmistakably different from those measured in Egypt and Nubia. The Jordanian values are lower than the Nile Valley values. Aridity was mentioned in the case of Nubia as a possible cause for such high nitrogen isotopic ratios, as was the hypothesis of freshwater fish consumption offered. Currently, lack of data from other areas of Jordan limits the interpretation of nitrogen isotopic values from North Jordan. As $\delta^{15}N$ values can reflect variables linked to both environment and diet, a baseline of such data, both human and faunal, is needed to help discriminate between possible causes.

Preliminary Conclusions and Future Work

The isotopic values from Bronze Age and Late Roman-Byzantine Tell Ya'amun and from Byzantine Khirbet Yajuz suggest that the individuals in the samples were homogenous in their access to protein sources. Even if these individuals were from different social backgrounds this seems not to have affected their access to such resources. Another question raised by these data regards the diachronic continuity in human diet over more than 2000 years at Tell Ya'amun. The skeletal remains of cattle, sheep and goat collected at this site may shed light on the environmental factors that could be responsible for the absence of change over time in the dietary patterns. Similarly, the discrepancies observed between the north of Jordan and the Nile Valley will be better interpreted when faunal isotopic data become available. Tests will be performed to establish if the differences between Bronze Age and Late Roman-Byzantine Tell Ya'amun, and between Tell Ya'amun and Khirbet Yajuz during Late Antiquity, are statistically significant.

Future work is aimed to collect samples and produce data from other Late Roman and/or Byzantine sites from north Jordan, including another agricultural settlement in North Jordan, Sa'ad, and the big city of Jerash. Data from Pella and Tell es-Sa'idiyeh, on the other hand, may reflect the ecological features of the Jordan Valley, as well as differences related to the geographical location and aspects of the economy.

Acknowledgements

Thanks go to my supervisors Dr Gundula Müldner and Prof Steven Mithen, to Prof. Bill Finlayson, and CBRL staff in Amman, to Prof. Mahmoud El-Najjar, Dr Abdulla Al-Shorman, Mr Mohammad Al-Rousan and Mr Ammar Al-Obiedat of Institute of Archaeology and Anthropology of Yarmouk University, Irbid, Jordan, to Prof Jerome Rose of the University of Arkansas, USA, to Dr Lutfi Khalil of the Department of Archaeology of the University of Jordan, Amman, and to the Department of Antiquities of Jordan, for access to the skeletal material. I would like to thank Leverhulme Trust for funding.

References

Al-Shorman, A. 2004. 'Stable carbon isotope analysis of human tooth enamel from the Bronze Age cemetery of Ya'amoun in Northern Jordan', *Journal of Archaeological Science* **31**, 1693–1698.

Ambrose, S. H. 1993. 'Isotopic analysis of palaeodiets: methodological and interpretative considerations', in Sandford, M. K. (ed.) *Investigation of Ancient Human Tissue: Chemical Analysis in Anthropology* (Langthorne), 59–130.

Anderson, J. D. 1998. 'The impact of Rome on the periphery: the case of Palestina – Roman Period (63BCE–324CE)', in Levy, T. E. (ed.) *The Archaeology of Society in the Holy Land* (London), 446–468.

Bocherens, H. and Drucker, D. 2003. 'Trophic level isotopic enrichment of carbon and nitrogen in bone collagen: case studies from recent and ancient terrestrial ecosystems', *International Journal of Osteoarchaeology* **13**, 46–53.

El-Najjar, M., Rose, J. C., Atallah, N., Turshan, N., Khasawneh, N. and Burke, D. L. 2001. 'First season of excavation at Ya'mun (1999)', *Annual of the Department of Antiquities of Jordan* **45**, 413–417.

Freeman, P. 2001. 'Roman Jordan', in Macdonald, B., Adams, R. and Bienkowski, P. (eds) *The Archaeology of Jordan* (Sheffield), 427–459.

Goodman, A. H., Dufour, D. L. and Pelto, G. H. 2000. *Nutritional Anthropology: Biocultural Perspectives on Food and Nutrition* (Mountain View).

Heaton, T. H. E., Vogel, J. C., La Chevallerie, G. V. and Collet, G. 1986. 'Climatic influence on the isotopic composition of bone nitrogen', *Nature* **322**, 822–823.

Iacumin, P., Bocherens, H., Chaix, L. and Marioth, A. 1998. 'Stable carbon and nitrogen isotopes as dietary indicators of ancient Nubian populations (Northern Sudan)', *Journal of Archaeological Science* **25**, 293–301.

Iacumin, P., Bocherens, H., Mariotti, A. and Longinelli, A. 1996. 'An isotopic palaeoenvironmental study of human skeletal remains from the Nile Valley', *Palaeogeography, Palaeoclimatology, Palaeoecology* **126**, 15–30.

Khalil, L. 1998. 'University of Jordan excavations at Khirbat Yajuz', *Annual of the Department of Antiquities of Jordan* **42**, 457–472.

Macdonald, B., Adams, R. and Bienkowski, P. 2001. *The Archaeology of Jordan* (Sheffield).

Macumber, P. G. 2001. 'Evolving landscape and environment in Jordan', in Macdonald, B., Adams, R. and Bienkowski, P. (eds) *The Archaeology of Jordan* (Sheffield), 1–30.

Oleson, J. P. 2001. 'Water supply in Jordan through the ages', in Macdonald, B., Adams, R. and Bienkowski, P. (eds.) *The Archaeology of Jordan* (Sheffield), 603–614.

Patrich, J. 1998. 'Church, state and transformation of Palestine – The Byzantine period (324–640 CE)', in Levy, T. E. (ed.) *The Archaeology of Society in the Holy Land* (London), 470–487.

Philip, G. 2001. 'The Early Bronze I–III Ages', in Macdonald, B., Adams, R. and Bienkowski, P. (eds.) *The Archaeology of Jordan* (Sheffield), 163–232.

Richards, M. P., Pearson, J. A., Molleson, T. I., Russell, N. and Martin, L. 2003. 'Stable isotope evidence of diet at Neolithic Çatalhöyük, Turkey', *Journal of Archaeological Science* **30**, 67–76.

Rose, J. C., El-Najjar, M. and Burke, D. L. in press. 'Trade and acquisition of wealth in rural Late Antique North Jordan', *Studies in the History and Archaeology of Jordan*.

Schoeninger, M. J., DeNiro, M. J. and Tauber, H. 1983. 'Stable nitrogen isotope ratios of bone collagen reflect marine and terrestrial components of prehistoric human diet', *Science* **220**, 1381–1383.

Schwarcz, H. P., Dupras, T. L. and Fairgrieve, S. I. 1999. '^{15}N enrichment in the Sahara: in search of a global relationship', *Journal of Archaeological Science* **26**, 629–636.

Schwarcz, H. P. and Schoeninger, M. J. 1991. 'Stable isotope analysis in human nutritional ecology', *Yearbook of Physical Anthropology* **34**, 283–321.

Sealy, J. 2001. 'Body tissue chemistry and palaeodiet', in Brothwell, D. R. and Pollard, A. M. (eds) *Handbook of Archaeological Sciences* (Chichester), 269–279.

Smith, B. N. and Epstein, S. 1971. 'Two categories of ^{13}C/^{12}C ratios for higher plants', *Plant Physiology* **47**, 380–384.

Suleiman, E. 1996. 'A short note on the excavations of Yajuz 1994–1995', *Annual of the Department of Antiquities of Jordan* **40**, 457–463.

Thompson, A. H., Chaix, L. and Richards, M. P. 2007. 'Stable isotopes and diet in Ancient Kerma, Upper Nubia (Sudan)', *Journal of Archaeological Science* **35** (2), 376–387.

Thompson, A. H., Richards, M. P., Shortland, A. and Zakrzewski, S. R. 2005. 'Isotopic palaeodiet studies of Ancient Egyptian fauna and humans', *Journal of Archaeological Science* **32**, 451–463.

Van Klinken, G. J., Richards, M. P. and Hedges, R. E. M. 2000. 'An overview of causes for stable isotope variations in past human European populations: environmental, ecophysiological, and cultural effects', in Ambrose, S. H. and Katzenberg, M. A. (eds) *Biogeochemical Approaches to Paleodietary Analysis* (New York), 39–63.

Watson, P. 2001. 'The Byzantine period', in Macdonald, B., Adams, R. and Bienkowski, P. (eds) *The Archaeology of Jordan* (Sheffield), 461–502.

Wiessner, P. 1996. 'Introduction: food, status, culture and nature', in Wiessner, P. and Schiefenhövel, W. (eds) Food and the Status Quest: An Interdisciplinary Perspective (Oxford), 1–18.

Website 1. www.waterlifecivilisation.org.

Feasting and Subsistence in Early Medieval Ireland and Wales: An Examination of the Literary and Archaeological Evidence

Anne Sassin,
University of Nottingham

Introduction
The social practice of feasting amongst the early Christian Celts is a highly contentious subject, most understanding of the situation being based on ambiguous literary evidence. Some of the earliest allusions to the social organization of early medieval Ireland come from the detailed law tracts of the seventh and eighth centuries, but it is sometimes difficult to determine how much they describe reality and how much an idealized world, as well as how much they reflect contemporary rather than older practices. Heroic sagas frequently mention feasts and, despite some fantastic elements, also reflect important aspects of society, including the concept of a 'hero' and his status at a feast. This has been fostered in the literature of other cultures, such as Homeric Greece, the Anglo-Saxon world (i.e. Beowulf) and Wales where similar hierarchical cultures functioning through clientship seem to have operated (Laing 2006, 16-18; Charles Edwards 1993, 477). Attempts to correlate historical information with the archaeological evidence have proved difficult and thus there is a need to adopt an integrated approach to the subject.

A widespread body of documentary evidence, supported in some measure by archaeological data, exists for the importance of feasting in Celtic society in Ireland and Wales in the early medieval period. Although there are many problems with the sources and their interpretation, cumulatively they point to a long-established European tradition, as well as various divergences between the Irish and Welsh feast, discrepancies concerning the halls in which they took place, and some oddities surrounding the social significance of cattle.

Feasting in Ireland
Society in early Christian Ireland functioned smoothly through clientship, in which the lord would hand over a 'gift' in exchange for defined dues, usually measured in cattle, for which the client would give such items as meat and cheese as well as physical labour (Laing 2006, 16). Besides military duty and raiding, these free clients carried out their obligations to their lord by providing the food-rents which enabled the lord to hold

feasts in return (Kelly 1998, 357). Both seasonal (e.g. 'the feast of Samain') and inaugural feasts were held, as well as those significant in the Church calendar, such as Easter (Kelly 1998, 359). Additionally, documentary and archaeological evidence suggest that music and the bardic narration of heroic and mythical tales were key components of Celtic feasting events. The most famous of the mythic sequences was the *Táin bó Cúailnge*, which was part of the Ulster Cycle and set in a mythical past, which concerned a war fought over the much-admired 'Brown Bull of Cooley' (Laing 2006, 27-28). Though the oldest written version of the text dates to the twelfth century, Jackson (1964, 48, 52) has suggested that the story reflects a much earlier (second century BC to fourth century AD) state of affairs: presumably the lack of Roman intervention allowed some Iron Age La Tène traditions to pass into this Early Christian literature.

What can be inferred about the classic feasting 'heroic society' portrayed in the Ulster Cycle and the provisions mentioned in the feasting scenes? Cakes of flour and honey are cited, but the chief food served seems to have been meat: beef and veal but most of all pork. Pigs were either cooked in cauldrons or roasted whole, and the best carcass was reserved for the chief hero to carve. This 'Champion's Portion' was literally a bone of contention, as several individuals could demand the privilege. If an opponent could not be put down with words, it might come to blows and even death; for although weapons were hung upon the wall when seated, they were never too far away (Jackson 1964, 21, 22).

Other sources make clear that the staple Irish diet consisted of bread and milk, with persons of higher rank enjoying a greater quantity and variety of meat (Kelly 1998, 316–319). The menu at royal feasts seems to have been very straightforward: roast or boiled meat and bread with mead and/or beer. Beer was frequently cited as a drink of social importance, for as the *Críth Gablach* states, a king who could not ensure beer every Sunday was not a proper ruler (Kelly 1998, 332). While the highest status guests received the best cuts of meat (e.g. the haunch), others received inferior pieces befitting their respective ranks (Kelly 1998, 359). Food was served on either a wooden platter or table, and drinks in wooden mugs and goblets, or in the case of the higher ranking, decorated drinking horns (Kelly 1998, 323).

Interestingly, parallels to the Irish practice can be found in Celtic Iron Age feasting on the continent, especially in the Celtic ethnography of the Stoic philosopher and historian Poseidonius. His work was often quoted in later sources, including the third-century AD instructive passage on Celtic food and drink by Athenaeus, which describes the 'occasional Celtic practice of single combat at meals' that sometimes led to death, as in the dispute over the 'hero's portion' mentioned above (Tierney 1960, 189, 201–202). Athenaeus further described the Celts as sitting on the dried grass for their meals, which were served on low tables, usually in a circle with the 'most influential man' in the centre, and one common cup passed around. While the drink of the wealthy was imported wine, the lower classes drank wheaten beer. Guests at the assembly exchanged jars of wine and gifts of silver and gold. One way for a leader to win popular favour was to prepare 'so great a quantity of food that for many days all who wished could enter and enjoy the feast prepared' (Tierney 1960, 247–248).

Exactly why the feasting traditions of Ireland and the continental Iron Age Celtic tribes were so similar is difficult to determine. The traditional interpretation is that both cultures were essentially the same. The study of Ireland's Iron Age background is complicated due to the debate over the extent of La Tène influence and the extent of relations with the Roman world. One school of thought maintains that the early medieval Celts were descendants from La Tène immigrants who introduced Celtic language and art forms from the continent around the third century BC. An alternative view argues that there is continuity of population and culture from earlier prehistory, with some influence from neighbouring La Tène societies. Though recent studies have provided clear evidence for contact with the Roman World, they have found little to suggest an intrusion of early Iron Age 'Celtic' settlers. Indeed, it now seems that the flourishing culture with major ritual centres which came to an end around the end of the millennium BC in Ireland was 'native' (Raftery 1994, 226–228), later passing into early medieval mythology and being reflected in later literature. Laing (2006, 272), amongst others, has speculated that this literature drew on a distant Iron Age memory but analyses of some material culture (e.g. swords) may show them to be much later, as the motifs may be better suited to the Viking Age rather than the La Tène period (Mallory 1982, 107). If this is the case, it seems likely that the common traditions are rooted in common Indo-European social organization.

Feasting in Wales

Feasting is also a prominent feature of the Welsh *Gododdin* poem, a lament to the fallen whose loyalty was bought through the hospitality of the mead-feast. Traditionally it was thought to have been composed in the sixth century by the poet Aneirin (e.g Jackson 1969, 58; Jarman 1988), but its linguistic elements have led some scholars (e.g. Dumville 1988) to see it as a twelfth-century composition, though presumably still reflecting early medieval feasting practices (De Vegvar 1995, 83). Throughout the poem 'good living' through feasting and drinking is the subject of consistent references, the arena being unsurprisingly the great hall, lit by tapers and well-fed fires, where the place of honour was 'at the end of the couch' (Jackson 1969, 34, 116). Although horns are the primary drinking vessel mentioned, glass tumblers are also described, with mead and wine the most frequently cited drinks. Interestingly, there is no mention of food as in the Irish sources, a situation akin to that seen in Anglo-Saxon literature (Maggenis 1999). One of the most informative lines, 'the pale mead was their feast and it was their poison', does not seem to refer to drunken stupor, but rather to how the men had risked their lives to earn it. This makes the recurrent mention of the hero 'earning his mead, paying for his mead and deserving his mead' a figure of speech for earning his bread, lodgings and weapons by performing his duty, and sometimes dying for it (Jackson 1969, 34–37).

Feasting and Subsistence

There seems no doubt that increasing contact between Ireland and Roman Britain from the late third century onwards, including Irish raiders and the establishment of settlements in Dyfed and north Wales, was instrumental in cultural exchange (Edwards 1990, 4–5); however, there is comparatively little evidence for Anglo-Saxon influence on Ireland except for art and ecclesiastical affairs (Laing 2006, 278), despite definite echoes of Anglo-Saxon feasting customs, as in Beowulf (Jackson 1969, 35–37). This makes it difficult to determine where precisely the origins lie, and whether Welsh feasting is echoed more in customs to the east in England or west across the Irish Sea; however the Irish parallels and divergences are certainly noteworthy.

Drinking Vessels

The social connotations behind drinking and alcohol consumption have already been mentioned, as it was an obligation of the upper social orders to provide vessels for consumption. Gift exchange established new socio-political relationships and reinforced old ones, with items such as imported vessels being used to associate the king's entourage with the highest social levels (Mytum 1992, 266–7). Élite drinking horns, usually represented archaeologically only by their metal terminals and fittings, are often listed amongst the possessions of the wealthy. Their magical capabilities, such as providing a limitless source of drink or transforming lesser liquids (e.g. brine) into more choice beverages, notably wine, are often mentioned (De Vegvar 1995, 81–82). Individuals of high status often named their horns, which were frequently composed of expensive materials, such as gold, and carried rich zoomorphic decoration. Slightly less privileged individuals owned horns with simpler terminals, such as the knob-shaped one at Clonmore, Co. Carlow or wooden ones such as that at Ballinderry 1, Co. Westmeath. It is interesting that no horns or fittings have been found in Wales, despite their frequent citation (De Vegvar 1995, 83). Whereas in Irish sources the horn itself is worthy of exchange, in Welsh literature the emphasis was more on the contents: a variety of both vessels and beverages are described. Specific references to drinking horns seem to be concentrated later in the twelfth and thirteenth centuries, with a common term *meddgorn* or 'mead-horn' implying that mead was the horn's primary beverage of choice, despite the *Gododdin's* recognition of other alcohol in this context (De Vegvar 1995, 85). Glass vessels figure more prominently in the Welsh poetry, though in both Ireland and Wales they represent Roman and later Merovingian and Carolingian industries (Bourke 1994, 163). Evidence from the high-status site of Dinas Powys in Wales certainly indicates fine drink consumption, with broken vessels being recovered from the 'hall' structure and the middens (Campbell 2000, 34–36, 40).

Halls

As far as the setting of the feast itself, excavated hall structures in Ireland and Britain bear little similarity to the impressive buildings suggested by the literature, which describes large thatched or shingled timber halls as well as smaller domed buildings of wattle and wicker (Laing 2006, 51). No halls have been identified for early Christian Ireland but for the rest of Celtic Britain archaeological evidence suggests that they consisted of one main dwelling with a few subsidiary barns. This is perhaps best exemplified by Cadbury Castle in Somerset where post-holes indicate a double-square plan with 'open-book' gables and partition within, measuring approximately 20 by 9.15 meters (Alcock 1995). Other possible timber halls have been found in northern England and Scotland, as well as at Dinas Powys, where the 'hall' is dubiously based on supposed eaves drips (Laing 2006, 52).

The apparent lack of identifiable halls in Ireland could be due to difficulties in interpreting timber structures, especially as total excavation is rarely carried out at ringforts and so sufficient ground plans are not recovered, as for instance at Rathmullan, Co. Down (Lynn 1981–2). Even structures of more substantial construction (e.g. clay and stone) are problematic to interpret because, until around the eighth century, dwellings were round rather than rectilinear, unfitting for the plan that would be expected for a hall, such as the square structure at Whitefort, Drumaroad, Co. Down (Waterman 1956; Edwards 1990, 22–23, 25).

Insight into non-ecclesiastical buildings for the period is complicated further by historical references and contemporary representations, the evidence rendered questionable by problems with translations and obvious descriptive exaggerations (Murray 1979, 81, 86). We know that grand residences of the period could be circular, such as the palace of Maeve at Cruachan described in the *Táin bó Fráich* but Jackson's (1964, 20) general reference to and interpretation of a similarly large wooden-framed building with carved and decorated pillars is vague in its ground plan. The bronze, silver and gold adornments on the pillars of the palace of Maeve may certainly be an embellishment to the standard, more basic form, yet the centrally placed hearths described are appropriate for a high-status hall setting (Murray 1979, 87). Similarly descriptions of the *imdai* ('compartment boxes' reserved for individual heroes) around the walls, which were probably curtained off for sleep at night, seem realistic (Murray 1979, 92–93; Jackson 1964, 20–21). Whether the Irish hall was definitely rectangular is hard to conclude, for although detailed 'plans' appear in both the twelfth-century *Book of Leinster* and later *Book of Lecan* of the 'Banqueting Hall' of Tara (the *Teach Miodhchuarta*) a literal interpretation might be misleading: the intended purpose of the plans was probably to illustrate the order of social grades listed. The fact that such images are more likely portrayals of twelfth-century features leaves questions concerning the form of early halls unanswered (Murray 1979, 93–94).

Cattle

In Irish society, the importance of cattle can be summarized as follows: 'land was measured in terms of the cows it could maintain, legal compensation was reckoned in terms of cattle, a man's standing in society was determined by his wealth of cattle, and cattle raiding was a recognized form of warfare and adventure for young nobles' (Ó Corráin 1972, 53). On the basis of evidence from literature and faunal remains, we know that the Irish economy was primarily pastoral, as it was in other Celtic regions, and that cattle were the dominant domesticate: on average cattle comprise 46 per cent of assemblages dating to after AD 400, and indeed, at Cahercommaun ringfort the figure was as high as 97 per cent (Ó Corráin 1976, 569; Laing 2006, 66–67). These figures are similar to those for Scotland but in Wales cattle are less well represented, their accounting for 37 per cent of assemblages, secondary to the pig bones on site (*ca.* 45 per cent). It should be noted, however, that these Welsh data derive from a single site (Dinas Powys) and so the sample is unlikely to be representative of the wider situation (Laing 2006, 66–67).

It is known that successful cattle-raids could demonstrate a ruler's political and military power (Kelly 1998, 28). Animals were often attributed with supernatural qualities and this, combined with their usefulness as suppliers of marrow, hides, tallow, horns and dung, encouraged people to own as many as possible, even where they began to compete with humans for food supplies (Kelly 1998, 53–57; Mytum 1992, 204). Faunal evidence suggests that cattle were kept for dairy produce as well as for meat (Laing 2006, 66) and, given that dairying was a more effective protein producer (McCormick 1983, 253), it is not surprising that the milch cow was a common form of payment (Kelly 1998, 27). Indeed, dairying may even have been the catalyst for giving cattle an essential role in the economy at the beginning of the Early Christian period (McCormick 1995, 35).

With this socio-economic prominence, cattle might be expected to figure to some degree in early Celtic art. Ox-heads of various forms were frequent in the pre-Roman Iron Age but as their economic importance supposedly increased (*ca.* sixth century), their prominence in Irish art almost disappeared (Laing and Laing 1992, 11, 117). It is true that 'Dark Age' art is considered less elaborate than what followed, but even with the 'Golden Age' of the eighth century this scarcity continued. Many early Irish gospel-books do contain the calf evangelist symbol of Saint Luke (Kelly 1998, 33) but this icon has Christian roots unaffected by insular influence. Other common animals appear in manuscript illuminations, such as in the Book of Kells, and are used mostly for symbolic purposes (Laing and Laing 1992, 146). This is a strange phenomenon, especially when considering the Pictish preference for everyday depictions, animal and hunting scenes (Carrington 1996, 459–468) versus the scriptural scenes clearly favoured amongst the Irish (Laing and Laing 1992, 170–172).

Pigs and Other Animals

Domestic fowl would presumably have been a suitable choice at feasts but they are poorly represented on archaeological sites and are not mentioned in the law codes until the seventh century. Similarly, while hunting features in the literature as an élite pursuit, the remains of game animals are also scarce on archaeological sites (Laing 2006, 69–70).

Pigs, however, are archaeologically abundant, their remains accounting for *ca.* 31 per cent of all animals represented in assemblages. As most seem to have been slaughtered before maturity, this suggests that they were primarily kept for meat (Laing 2006, 67). Certainly the flesh of pigs, in particular salted pork, was highly favoured (Kelly 1998, 336). Their obvious preference in the literature over cattle as the choice meat of the feast may be due to the alternate use of cows (i.e. dairying), although instances reflecting traditions in pre-dairying societies would not take this into account. It is interesting that at Dinas Powys pig remains predominate (Laing 2006, 67), perhaps suggesting that feasting was a regular activity at this site, and this contrast with the Irish evidence and comparably less evidence for the significance of cattle in Wales raises questions, even if no inferences can be made.

Conclusions

The major problem in assessing Celtic feasting practices is the lack of excavation and documented evidence for early Christian Wales, especially compared to Ireland. Without additional historical and archaeological data it is impossible to say whether cattle played less of a role in Welsh society than in Irish, or if cattle were represented less at feasts due to their value as milk producers. The same lack of defining evidence for pigs makes their role in the Irish versus the Welsh feast setting equally uncertain. With so many theories concerning the historicity of tales like the Ulster Cycle and *Gododdin*, it is similarly difficult to pinpoint the origins of various components of the feast and whether or not they had a common source. In the absence of more detailed archaeological plans of potential feast 'halls' in Ireland, it will also not be known how accurate the literary descriptions are. Yet the negative evidence of their known existence when compared to British examples stands out as highly intriguing.

Though it is difficult to state anything concise in such instances when the evidence is dubious in its interpretation, the underlying theme is a deep-rooted European tradition behind various aspects of the Celtic feast, with an assortment of regional deviations apparent in Britain and Ireland. However, there certainly appears to be room for further research, as well as reassessment of the existing material, in order for the dubieties to be addressed.

References

Alcock, L. 1995. *Cadbury Castle, Somerset: The Early Medieval Archaeology* (Cardiff).
Bourke, E. 1994. 'Glass vessels of the first nine centuries AD in Ireland', *Journal of the Royal Society of Antiquaries of Ireland* **124**, 163–209.
Campbell, E. 2000. 'A review of glass vessels in western Britain and Ireland AD 400–800', in Price, J. (ed.) *Glass in Britain and Ireland AD 350–1100* (London), 33–46.
Carrington, A. 1996. 'The horseman and the falcon: mounted falconers in Pictish sculpture', *Proceedings of the the Society of Antiquaries of Scotland* **126**, 459–468.
Charles-Edwards, T. M. 1993. *Early Irish and Welsh Kinship* (Oxford).

De Vegvar, C. N. 1995. 'Drinking horns in Ireland and Wales: documentary sources', in Bourke, C. (ed.) *From the Isles of the North: Early Medieval Art in Ireland and Britain* (Belfast), 81–87.

Dumville, D. 1988. 'Early Welsh poetry, problems in historicity' in Roberts, B. F (ed.) *Early Welsh Poetry: Studies in the Book of Aneurin* (Aberystwyth), 1–16.

Edwards, N. 1990. *The Archaeology of Early Medieval Ireland* (London).

Jackson, K. H. 1964. *The Oldest Irish Tradition: A Window on the Iron Age* (Cambridge).

Jackson, K. H. 1969. *The Gododdin: The Oldest Scottish Poem* (Edinburgh).

Jarman, A. O. H. 1988. *Aneirin: Y Gododdin, Britain's Oldest Heroic Poem* (Llandysul).

Kelly, F. 1998. *Early Irish Farming* (Dublin).

Laing, L. 2006. *The Archaeology of Celtic Britain and Ireland, c. AD 400–1200* (Cambridge).

Laing, L. and Laing, J. 1992. *Art of the Celts* (London).

Lynn, C. J. 1981-2. 'The excavation of Rathmullan, a raised rath and motte in Co. Down' *Ulster Journal of Archaeology* **44–5**, 65–171.

Mallory, J. P. 1982. 'The sword of the Ulster Cycle', in Scott, B. (ed.) *Studies on Early Ireland: Essays in Honour of M. V. Duignan* (Belfast), 99–114.

Magennis, H. 1999. *Anglo-Saxon Appetites: Food and Drink and Their Consumption in Old English and Related Literature* (Bodmin).

McCormick, F. 1983. 'Dairying and beef production in early Christian Ireland: the faunal evidence', in Reeves-Smith, T. and Hammond, F. (eds) *Landscape Archaeology in Ireland* (Oxford), 253–267.

McCormick, F. 1995. 'Cows, ringforts and the origins of early Christian Ireland', *Emania* **13**, 33–37.

Murray, H. 1979. 'Documentary evidence for domestic buildings in Ireland, c. 400–1200 in the light of archaeology', *Medieval Archaeology* **23**, 81–97.

Mytum, H. 1992. *The Origins of Early Christian Ireland* (London).

Ó Corráin, D. 1972. *Ireland Before the Normans* (Dublin).

Ó Corráin, D. 1976. 'Ireland c. 800: aspects of society', in Ó Corráin, D. (ed.) *A New History of Ireland* (Oxford), 549–608.

Raftery, B. 1994. *Pagan Celtic Ireland: The Enigma of the Irish Iron Age* (London).

Tierney, J. J. 1960. 'The Celtic ethnography of Posidonius', *Proceedings of the Royal Irish Academy* **60**, 189–275.

Waterman, D. M. 1956. 'The excavation of a house and souterrain at Whitefort, Drumarood, Co. Down', *The Ulster Journal of Archaeology* **19**, 73–86.

Figure 14.1. Table illustrating different periods through time and space in both the Near East and the Aegean, based on Roaf (1990, 8–9) and Dickinson (1994, 19).

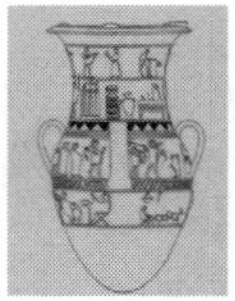

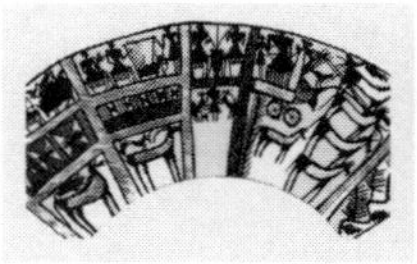

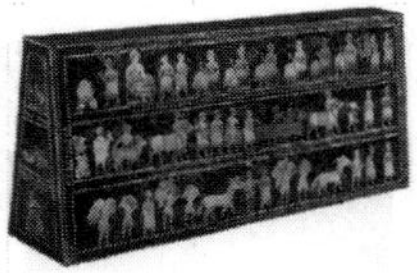

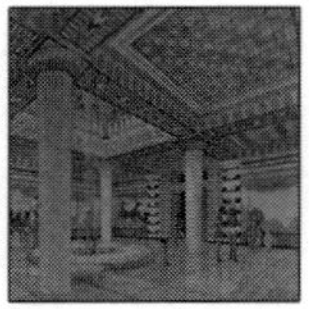

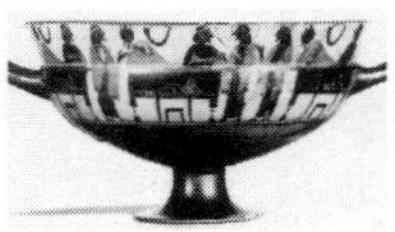

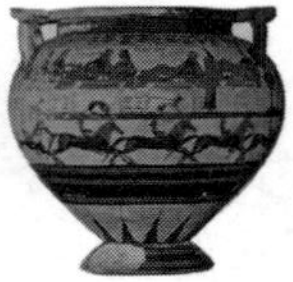

The Origins of the Archaic Greek *Symposium*: Internal Developments and Near Eastern Influences

Karin Schuitema,
Leiden University

Introduction

When scholars of the nineteenth century started recognizing parallels between Homeric epics and Near Eastern cuneiform texts, the concept of an isolated Greece began to dissolve (Burkert 2004). Cultural interaction, which must have exchanged objects as well as ideas, is now identifiable from the Early Bronze Age to the 'Orientalizing Period' and later Archaic period (spanning a date range from *ca.* 3200 BC to 480 BC, see Fig. 14.1) through a study of objects, but is difficult to identify in the social developments in the Aegean. Material remains and texts, however, suggest that traditions associated with feasting reflect hierarchical aspects of both societies while simultaneously revealing an ideological exchange visible in the Aegean and Near East.

This paper presents a diachronic study of the ancient feast in the Aegean areas of mainland Greece, Crete, the Near Eastern areas of Mesopotamia, the Levant, and Anatolia. As an important intermediary between East and West, Cyprus is also considered (the geographical range and sites considered in this paper are shown in figure 14.2). I focus particularly on Archaic Greek *symposia,* a specific kind of feast – involving communal drinking after a meal (the *deipnon*), during which participants reclined instead of sitting – that appeared in Greece around the end of the seventh century BC and utilized many luxurious oriental customs. By comparing feasting traditions in the Aegean and Near East, I aim to trace the origins of the Archaic Greek *symposium* and investigate whether its social implications were adopted from the Near East.

This study builds upon previous research that has considered similar issues (Matthäus 1999; Reade 1995) but, unlike previous work, this paper concentrates on the question of whether the social implications of feasts in the Aegean were adopted from the Near East along with the physical characteristics of these rituals and, if so, what were these social implications and what role did they play in Hellenic social discourse? I suggest that Near Eastern influences on Aegean feasting pre-date Archaic Greek *symposia* and that these influences are visible in certain aspects of Aegean feasts that continue from the Bronze Age into Archaic times.

Most previous studies of social change in Archaic Greek Society, such as the emergence of *symposia*, regarded these changes as separate developments, independent of Bronze and Early Iron Age practices (Murray 1983; Osborne 1996; Whitley 2001). McGovern (2003, 258), however, argues that the roots of a special wine-drinking

The Origins of the Archaic Greek Symposium

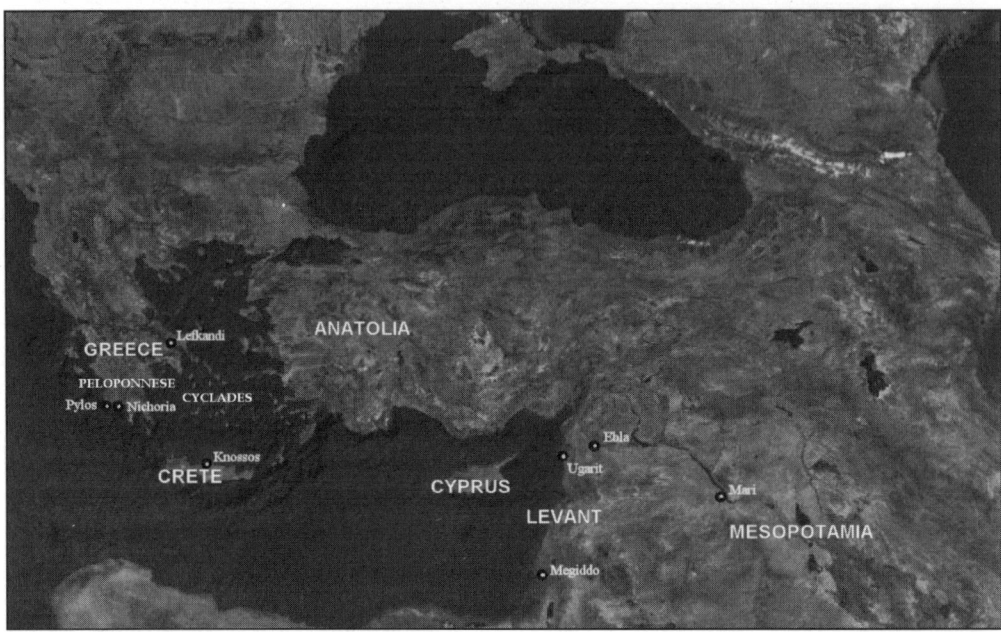

Figure 14.2. Map of the Aegean and the Near East with indications of the sites mentioned in the text.

ceremony similar to the Greek *symposium* can be traced back to the Middle Minoan Period (2160–1600 BC) and Mycenaean palace life. Crielaard (pers. comm.) advocates the possibility of continuity in feasting traditions from the Late Bronze to the Iron Age in the coastal areas of Anatolia and in Cyprus. I suggest that these areas were part of a 'feasting *koine*', that is, a communal feasting tradition.

In this paper I will consider material evidence of feasting, drawn from ethnographic observations, from the following categories: iconography, vessel assemblages, feasting locations, and furniture (Dietler and Hayden 2001). Each of these material groups has its own limitations. Iconographical representations, for instance, are often self-reflections or propaganda, displaying how a group sees itself rather than reality. Furthermore, not all scenes of people holding cups should be interpreted as representations of feasting, as identification of a 'feasting vessel' is often ambiguous (Dabney *et al.* 2004). Feasting locations are also difficult to identify, since not all architectural structures necessarily have *in-situ* deposits clearly associated with feasts. Locations can, however, sometimes be identified on the basis of specific architectural elements. Luxurious furniture, for example, although often found out of context or in burials, may indicate a feasting location.

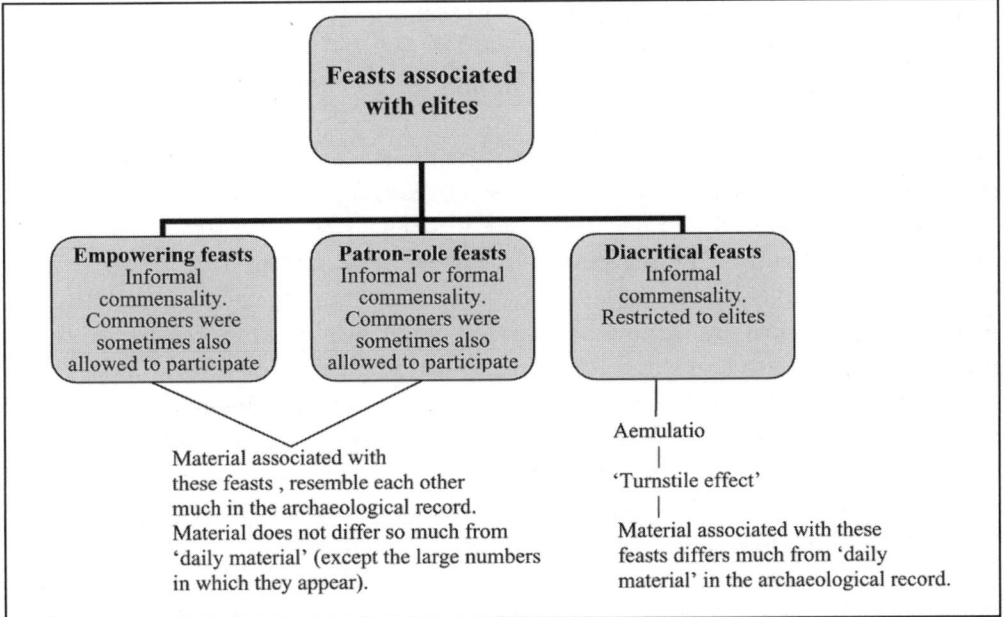

Figure 14.3. The three modes of élite feasts as distinguished by Dietler (2001, 81). Image courtesy of Michael Dietler.

Definition and Theoretical Classifications of Feasting

Recently, feasting has become a popular theme in archaeological studies examining the ways in which individuals and groups created and maintained their social positions (Ralph 2005). It is hard to give an unambiguous definition of feasting since this term is used to describe a wide range of practices (Dietler and Hayden 2001). Here, feasting is defined as a ritualized event, differing from daily consumption practices, in which an aggregation of people and communal consumption of food and drink are the most important aspects, along with a certain form of display (such as displaying status by drinking from elaborate cups or by displaying weapons on the walls of the dining space, or by wearing rich clothes). The term 'ritualized' in this definition is used to emphasize that consumption is not taking place solely for sustenance but is considered a facet of a greater social event (Clarke 2001, 145). Other activities are often observed in addition to these prerequisites, such as singing, dancing and discourse (Wiessner 2001, 117).

Classifying feasts as 'empowering,' 'patron-role,' or 'diacritical' (Fig. 14.3, and see Dietler 2001, 81) highlights distinctions and similarities between different feasting types. The different natures of feasts should not be over-generalized, however: their *emic* meaning, i.e. their culture-specific truth, and the way in which they present themselves in the archaeological record should not be ignored.

Exchanges Between Aegean and Near Eastern Feasts: A Feasting *Koine* from the Bronze to the Iron Age

I consider social drinking, which was common in the Near East by the late fourth/early third millennium BC, to be a direct ancestor of the *symposium*. This relationship is especially clear from Mesopotamian iconography where communal drinking scenes are an important theme (Viviani 2005). Most feasts in the early third millennium in Mesopotamia took place in temples and appear to have been associated with the disbursal of food rations. By the second half of the third millennium, however, feasts were more commonly held in palaces – the new centres of political organization – and their message was now one of royal prestige and power-display, a message echoed by the iconographic representations of feasting in this period (Schmandt-Besserat 2001).

Although the third millennium witnessed many changes in Mesopotamian feasting traditions, continuity can be demonstrated by the occasions warranting such practices, namely war, hunting, and the *kispu* ritual of venerating deceased ancestors (Reade 1995). It is possible that the *kispu* ritual was the progenitor of the *marzeah*, a special feast restricted to high-class landowning men, involving deity and ancestor worship as well as wine consumption (Carter 1995). Mentions of the term *marzeah* are visible in third millennium texts from Ebla, although no clear meaning can be inferred (McLaughlin 1991). The first unambiguous identifications of the *marzeah* as a feast are found in thirteenth-century BC texts from Ugarit (McGovern 2003).

Already in the late fourth and early third millennium BC, viticulture had spread from the Caucasus to Anatolia, Mesopotamia, and the Levant (McGovern 2003; Zettler and Miller 1996). Through the course of the third millennium, the drinking of wine instead of beer became important at élite gatherings, introducing a new element into prestigious social discourses. Around the middle of the third millennium BC these new elements of social interaction combined and were copied by Aegean élites via Southern Anatolia and Cyprus, becoming a so-called 'international style' of feasting (Zettler and Miller 1996). Meat consumption also seems to have been of considerable importance in this 'feasting *koine*,' with meat being prepared in cauldrons (Wright 2004). Such cauldrons, together with exotic drinking and pouring vessels, such as *rhyta*, spread from western and southern Anatolia, via Cyprus, to the Cyclades in the Early and Middle Bronze Age. They also appear in Crete (McGovern 2003).

Exchanges between the East and West became more frequent from the third to the second millennium BC. This continuous interaction affected feasting traditions in both regions. Paintings from the palace of Mari and ivories from Megiddo from the second millennium provide examples of iconography related to the *marzeah*, and are indicative of the type of feast most frequently represented in both images and texts from this period in the Near East. In the Levant especially, this material resembles contemporary evidence of the Mycenaean feast (e.g. in the Palace of Nestor, Pylos) in both style and subject matter. While similarities in iconography do not necessarily reflect similarities in actual performance, it is notable that depictions of the *marzeah* resemble those of Mycenaean feasting rituals not only in style and representation, but also in terms of their placement within central rooms of palatial complexes (Bendall 2004). The occasions on which a feast would be performed were also very similar: the veneration of a god or deceased ancestor, hunting, warfare, or a certain *rite de passage* (Wright 2004). Both the Levantine *marzeah* and Mycenaean feasts were held by a ruler in order to win the allegiance of élite citizenry, serving as both 'diacritical' and 'patron role feasts' simultaneously (Fig. 14.3). Indeed, it seems that social contacts and an appetite for distinguishing customs and exotic objects influenced élites in the Near East and the Aegean, which gave rise to similar feasting cultures. One possible difference between the Levantine *marzeah* and the Mycenaean feast, however, warrants mention. Status differences existed between the élites participating in the *marzeah*, as can be inferred from the Megiddo Ivory 160, where the size of drinking bowls corresponds with the proximity of the participant to the ruler (Yasur-Landau 2005). By contrast, status differences in the Mycenaean feast were de-emphasized by the use of simple standardized vessels by participants, many of which have been found in Mycenaean palaces (Dabney *et al.* 2004, 197–215; Fox and Harrell this volume), with only the host drinking from an elaborate vessel. Furthermore, participants in Mycenaean feasting representations are often depicted at the same scale and with similar attire, as on the *megaron* fresco from the Palace of Nestor, Pylos (Wright 2004).

Despite minor differences in ceremony, contacts between élites allowed an exchange of feasting-type vessels: *kraters, rhyta, situlae* and beak-spouted jars spread from the Near East into the Aegean, while Mycenaean *kraters* and stirrup jars were exported to the coastal parts of the Levant (Van Wijngaarden 1999). While imports to the Levant were certainly associated with drinking, it is unclear whether they were used in élite feasting or daily life. The importation of these vessels probably did not influence Near Eastern feasting practices. Instead, the shape and style of Mycenaean vessels were adapted to Levantine customs, just as Near Eastern furniture used in Aegean feasts – such as the campstool chair and the three-legged table, known from the famous 'Campstool Fresco' from Knossos (Wright 1996) – was adapted to conform to Aegean traditions.

The exchanges described above are closely related to *xenia* connections, i.e. relationships that tied élites from different areas together. This bi-directional influence was fuelled by *aemulatio*, or lower-class people, adopting certain objects and customs from élites. To keep above the masses, élites found new ways of expressing themselves, often through the adoption of exotic objects and foreign customs. Mutual adoptions inspired the creation of an élite feasting *koine* as an essential part of an upper-class lifestyle throughout the Aegean and the Eastern Mediterranean in the Late Bronze Age.

While evidence suggests continuity in Aegean feasting from the Bronze Age to the Iron Age, unambiguous evidence of feasting in 'Dark Age' Greece is scarce. Most of what we know about feasts in this period is derived from Homer's poems. Information taken from these poems must be treated with caution, however, as the society described by Homer is a mixture of the eighth/seventh century BC (Homer's own time), the tenth/ninth century BC, and the Bronze Age (*ca.* 1200 BC) (Antonaccio 1995; Crielaard 1995).

Iron Age sites can demonstrate how the presence or absence of a palace affected the role of feasting within a community and indicate whether certain aspects continued from the Bronze Age into the Early Iron Age. Suggestive material, however, is chronologically and regionally distinct, and expressions of feasting from the Bronze Age into the Early Iron Age differ with date, location and context. The sites considered have been selected because they were all major centres during their respective periods. Important Early Iron Age evidence is found at post-palatial Euboean sites, such as Xeropolis and Toumba in Lefkandi (Antonaccio 1995; Popham 1987). The settlement of Nichoria (Rapp *et al.* 1978) in western Messenia provides us, when compared to other Iron Age sites, with a detailed view of various feasting rituals circulating in Iron Age Greece. A comparison of feasting at these three sites suggests that feasts at post-palatial sites shared common characteristics not found at palatial centres. Post-palatial feasting seems to have operated on a smaller scale from that of the palaces and functioned as an expression of a less hierarchically-oriented group identity. Feasts from Xeropolis, Toumba and Nichoria, however, differed in their motivations, means of expression, and the kinds of bonds they created among the participants. The feasting at Xeropolis was centred within individual households rather than a single large-scale venue. Despite a seemingly modest scale, the prevalence of imported vessels and pictorial *kraters* indicates that Xeropolis feasting emphasized display. Contrary to the decentralized feasts at Xeropolis, the large size and central location of the feasts at Nichoria were probably inclusive and communally focused. The feasts held in the Toumba building at Lefkandi were likely based on establishing links with other élites through the projection of warrior ideologies, which is comparable with the late second/early first millennium BC *marzeah*. These examples indicate the variability and the multiple forms of feasting behaviour that existed in the Early Iron Age and reflect the need of post-palatial communities for various, nuanced forms of group unity and solidarity.

The spread of specific types of Near Eastern vessels from Anatolia into the Aegean, such as metal cauldrons and ram/lion-headed *situlae,* continued from the Bronze into the Iron Age (McGovern 2003). In the other direction, many Iron Age Greek vessels related to drinking and dining, like *oinochoe* and *amphora*, were imported into the Levant. Contacts became even more frequent during the eighth century BC (Luke 2003). The similarities between the Early Iron Age feasts in the Aegean and the early first millennium BC *marzeah* arose out of a combination of close contacts between East and West, and the fact that the early first millennium BC *marzeah* developed out of the second millennium BC *marzeah,* which resembled the Mycenaean feast. I suggest that many aspects of Early Iron Age feasts developed out of the Mycenaean feast, although their social functions differed. In both, a dominant persona hosted the feast in order to earn the allegiance of élites. In turn, the attending élites gain increased status through their participation.

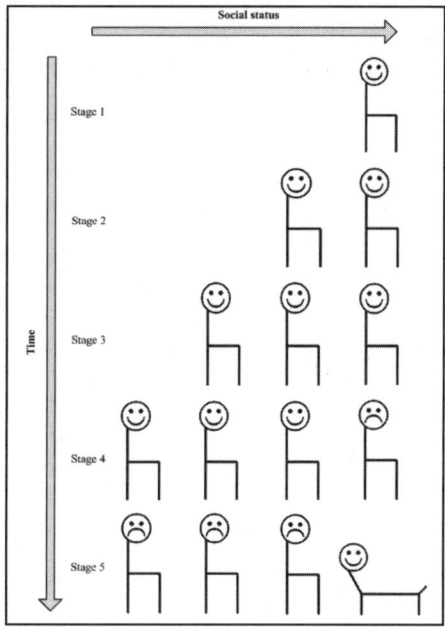

Figure 14.4. The concept of emulation related to the emergence of the reclining symposium in the Aegean. Horizontal axis: social status. Vertical axis: changes in feasting customs through time, showing the introduction of a new dining posture as a custom of distinction by higher groups (after Nieuwenhuyse 2006).

In the Archaic Period the *symposium* emerged as an important feast in the Aegean. Both the Early Iron Age feast, observable at Toumba, and the Archaic *symposium* consolidated reciprocal bonds between élites (*xenoi*). Various similarities existed between Iron Age feasts and Archaic *symposia*: consumption of food and drinks in company with other élites, the display of weapons on dining-room walls, and the use of prestigious drinking vessels to distinguish élites from the rest of the population. While the Early Iron Age feast served to create bonds between wealthy warrior classes, the emergence of *poleis* (city states) in the eighth century BC changed forever the dynamics of social hierarchy.

The emergence of a hoplite army allowed non-élite citizens to begin fulfilling warrior tasks that previously were the exclusive privilege of élites, but Archaic *symposia* were not used to form warrior groups. Instead, *symposia* of the Archaic Period provided a stage on which the upper class could distinguish itself from the common citizenry by its luxurious and lavish lifestyle. The élites placed themselves above the *polis* by identifying themselves as a class of internationally-élite figures (Crielaard 2003, 323). The *symposium* is, therefore, often regarded as a phenomenon of conspicuous consumption, completely separate from politics or the organization of the *polis*, with no direct economic, religious, or organizational purpose. Sometimes it is even regarded as an event opposing the *polis* ideology through its abundance and waste. Warrior

The Origins of the Archaic Greek Symposium

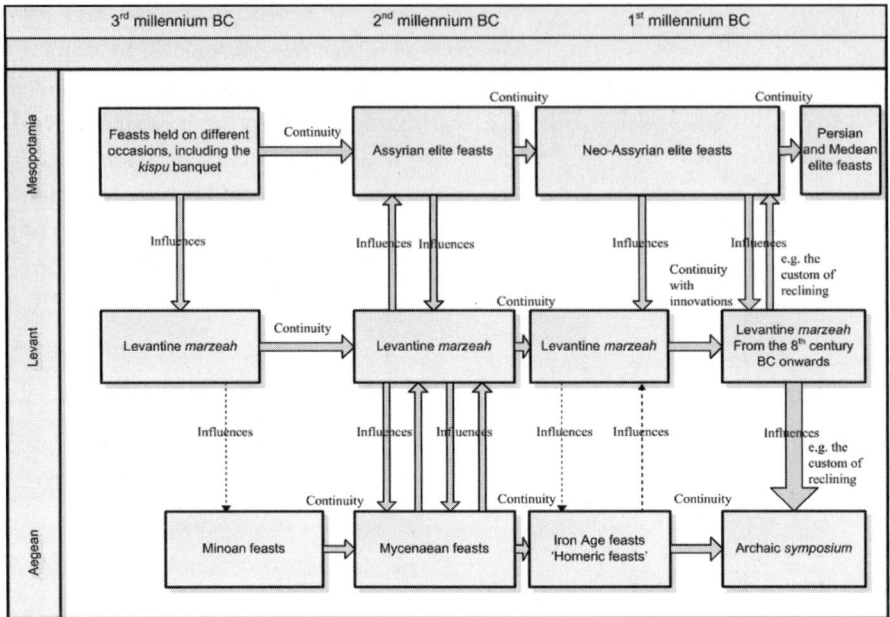

Figure 14.5. The development of and influences on the Archaic Greek symposium.

aspects, however, were still associated with élites and, therefore, present at the Archaic *symposia*. The ways in which élites distinguished themselves in the Archaic *symposium* may also have been influenced by the Near East. Greek élites, who had lost many of their political privileges, needed new symbols to distinguish themselves from the rest of the population. They found the answer by adopting many aspects of the luxurious lifestyle of Levantine élites. Exotic adoptions are closely related to emulation. This phenomenon implies vertical adoption of élite customs by people of lower status in society, due to which élites need to find new symbols to express their high status (see Fig. 14.4). An example of such an exotic adoption was the custom of reclining during a banquet, which came from the Near East, as can be inferred from prophetic texts and depictions of banquets on Syro-Phoenician bowls found in Cyprus (Stampolidis 2003, 344). The custom is present in the Levantine *marzeah* from the eighth century BC and communicated the idea of luxury. Greek élites adopted reclining somewhere around this time in order to identify themselves with high-status figures from the Near East, where this custom was the prerogative of kings and rulers (Crielaard 2003).

A common élite lifestyle in the Aegean and the Near East is therefore visible from the Bronze Age into the Archaic Period, with the most active interactions occurring during the Late Bronze Age and Orientalizing Period (see Fig. 14.5).

Conclusion

Many of the Near Eastern aspects in the Archaic Greek *symposium,* such as the custom of reclining, were adopted in the Orientalizing Period, but some, like the exclusion of all non-élites, originated from an earlier feasting *koine* within the area of the Near East and the Aegean, which itself had roots in social drinking that date back to the third millennium BC. The social function of the *symposium* should therefore be regarded as an internal development within Greece that reflects Aegean hierarchical dynamics of the Archaic Period by evoking luxurious exoticism commonly associated with the Near East (Schuitema 2007).

References

Antonaccio, C. M. 1995. '*Lefkandi and Homer*', in Andersen, Ø. and Bergen, M. D. (eds) *Homer's World: Fiction, Tradition, Reality* (Bergen), 5–28.

Bendall, L. M. 2004. 'Fit for a king? hierarchy, exclusion, aspiration and desire in the social structure of Mycenaean banqueting', in Halstead, P. and Barrett, J. C. (eds) *Food, Cuisine and Society in Prehistoric Greece* (Oxford), 105–35.

Bray, T. L. 2003. *The Archaeology and Politics of Food and Feasting in Early States and Empires* (New York).

Burkert, W. 2004. *Babylon, Memphis, Persepolis: Eastern Contexts of Greek Culture* (London).

Carter, J. B. 1995. 'Ancestor cult and the occasion of Homeric performance', in Carter J. B. and Morris S. P. (eds) *The Ages of Homer: A Tribute to Emily Vermeule* (Austin) 285–312.

Clarke, M. 2001. 'Akha feasting: an ethnoarchaeological perspective', in Dietler, M. and Hayden, B. (eds) *Feasts: Archaeological and Ethnographic Perspectives on Food, Politics and Power* (Washington), 144–167.

Crielaard, J. P. 1995. *Homeric Questions : Essays in Philology, Ancient History and Archaeology, Including the Papers of a Conference Organized by the Netherlands Institute at Athens (15 May 1993)* (Amsterdam).

Crielaard, J. P. 2003. 'Lyriek, materiële cultuur en identiteit in Archaïsch Oost-Griekenland', *Lampas* **36** (4), 60–84.

Dabney, M. K., Halstead, P. and Thomas, P. 2004. 'Mycenaean feasting on Tsoungiza at ancient Nemea', *Hesperia* **73** (2), 197–216.

Dickinson, O. 1994. *The Aegean Bronze Age* (Cambridge)

Dietler, M. and Hayden, B. 2001. *Feasts: Archaeological and Ethnographic Perspectives on Food, Politics and Power* (Washington)

Dietler, M. 2001. 'Theorizing the feasts: rituals of consumption, commensal politics, and power in African contexts', in Dietler, M. and Hayden, B. (eds) *Feasts: Archaeological and Ethnographic Perspectives on Food, Politics and Power* (Washington), 65–114.

Luke, J. 2003. *Ports of Trade: Al Mina and Geometric Greek pottery in the Levant* (Oxford).

Matthäus, H. 1999. 'Das griechische Symposion und der Orient', *Nürnberger Blätter zur Archäologie* **16**, 41–64.

McGovern, P. E. 2003. *Ancient Wine: The Research for the Origins of Viniculture* (Princeton).

McLauhlin, J. L. 1991. 'The Marzeah at Ugarit: a textual and contextual study', *Ugarit-Forschungen: Internationales Jahrbuch für die Altertumskunde Syrien-Palästinas* **23**, 265–282.

Murray, O. 1983. 'The symposium as social organisation', in Hägg, R. (ed.) *The Greek Renaissance of the Eighth Century B.C.: Tradition and Innovation* (Stockholm), 195–199.

Nieuwenhuyse, O. 2006. *Plain and Painted Pottery: The Rise of Late Neolithic Ceramic Styles on the Syrian and Northern Mesopotamian Plains* Unpublished PhD thesis, Leiden University.

Osborne, R. 1996. *Greece in the Making 1200–479 BC* (London).

Popham, M. 1987. 'Lefkandi and the Greek Dark Age', in Cunliffe, B. W. (ed.) *Origins: The Roots of European Civilisation* (London), 67–80.

Ralph, S. 2005. 'Eat, drink and be Roman? Feasting in later Iron Age and Early Roman Britain', in Ralph, S. (ed.) *Archaeological Review from Cambridge* **20** (2), 32–52.

Rapp, G. R., Aschenbrenner, S. E. and McDonald, W. A. 1978. *Excavations at Nichoria in Southwest Greece* (Minneapolis).

Reade, J. 1995. 'The symposion in ancient Mesopotamia: archaeological evidence', in Murray, O and Tecuşan, M. (eds) *In Vino Veritas* (London), 35–56.

Roaf, M. 1990. *Cultural Atlas of Mesopotamia and the Ancient Near East* (New York).

Schmandt-Besserat, D. 2001. 'Feasting in the Ancient Near East', in Dietler, M. and Hayden, B. *Feasts: Archaeological and Ethnographic Perspectives on Food, Politics and Power* (Washington), 391–403.

Schuitema, K. E. 2007. *In Pursuit of the Symposium: A Diachronic, Comparative Study on Feasting in the Aegean and the Near East*, Unpublished Masters thesis, Leiden University.

Stampolidis N. C. 2003. 'On the Phoenician presence in the Aegean', in Stampolidis N. C. and Karageorghis, V. (eds) *Sea Routes... From Sidon to Huelva. Interconnections in the Mediterranean 16th–6th c. BC* (Athens), 217–32.

Van Wijngaarden, G. J. M, 1999. *Use and Appreciation of Mycenaean Pottery Outside Greece : Contexts of LHI–LHIIIB Finds in the Levant, Cyprus and Italy* (London).

Viviani, M. T. 2005. 'The role of alcoholic beverages in Sumer and Akkad: an analysis of iconographic patterns (III Millennium)', *Aram Periodical* **17**, 1–50.

Whitley, J. 2001. *The Archaeology of Ancient Greece* (Cambridge).

Wiessner, P. 2001. 'Of feasting and value: Enga feasts in a historical perspective (Papua New Guinea)', in Dietler, M. and Hayden, B. *Feasts: Archaeological and Ethnographic Perspectives on Food, Politics, and Power*, (Washington), 115–143.

Wright, J. C. 1996. 'Empty cups and empty jugs: the social role of wine in Minoan and Mycenaean societies', in McGovern, P. E., Fleming, S. J. and Katz, S. H. (eds) *The Origins and History of Wine*, (Philadelphia), 287–309.

Wright, J. C. 2004. 'The Mycenaean Feast: an introduction', *Hesperia* **73** (2), 121–132.

Yasur-Landau, A. 2005. 'Old wine in new vessels: intercultural contact, innovation and Aegean, Canaanite and Philistine foodways', in Cohen, Y. and Yasur-Landau, A. (eds) *Journal of the Institute of Archaeology of Tel Aviv University* **32** (2), 168–191.

Zettler, R. L. and Miller, N. F. 1996. 'Searching for wine in the archaeological record of ancient Mesopotamia of the third and second millennia B.C.', in McGovern, P. E., Fleming, S. J. and Katz, S. H. (eds) *The Origins and Ancient History of Wine* (Philadelphia), 123–131.

Foodways as a Reflection of Cultural Identity in a Roman Frontier Province – Bridging the Gap from Theory to Material

Aviva Shuman,
University of Amsterdam

'Identity' is a word that is currently fashionable in archaeological circles, especially Roman studies; yet attempts to approach the subject through material culture have been of limited success. I believe this is, in part, because there is no common theoretical vocabulary for discussing the subject. For some, identity is simply another word for 'ethnicity'. Ethnicity is, without doubt, an aspect of identity but it can hardly be said to represent the whole picture. In Roman archaeology it seems that 'identity' is sometimes used to avoid the now unfashionable 'Romanization', but without resolving the issues inherent in that term. So where do we turn to find a theoretical vocabulary that we can use? The most logical place to look is within the social sciences where identity has been a part of the discourse within anthropology and sociology for decades. Although in much of Europe archaeology is regarded mainly as a historical discipline, it is not simply a study of the past; it is a study of people and societies in the past, and as such it is equally a social science. This is reflected in curricula in North America where archaeology is categorized as a daughter-discipline to anthropology. If we want to understand how identities are created, recreated and reflected in the material culture and depositional processes, social science is better equipped to provide us with models than history.

Defining identity is no easy task. Even looking at the common usage, the complexity of this term becomes clear. For example, *The American Heritage Dictionary* (Website 1) defines identity as both 'the set of behavioral or personal characteristics by which an individual is recognizable as a member of a group,' and 'the distinct personality of an individual regarded as a persisting entity; individuality'. Paradoxically, identity is both that which defines one as an individual, and that which connotes group membership. Given the complexity of identity, what do archaeologists mean when we use the term? In *The Archaeology of Identity*, Díaz-Andreu *et al.* (2005, 1) define it 'as individuals' identification with broader social groups on the basis of differences socially sanctioned as significant'. This helps us to narrow down the definition but it does not bring us closer to understanding how identities are formed, reformed and negotiated within societies. Identity is not a fixed quality, impervious to agency. People can play with the qualities that make them who they are, negotiating social fields and emphasizing certain aspects of identity while suppressing others, depending on the context. At the same time our world view and beliefs about our identity are shaped by our socialization at an early age. Bourdieu's practice theory has provided us with the useful concept of the *habitus*, most succinctly described as 'durable dispositions towards certain perceptions and practices…which can become part of an individual's sense of self at an early age, and which can be transported from one context to another' (Jones 1997, 88). It is this focus on practices that makes foodways an ideal lens through which to view identity.

According to sociologist Claude Fischler (1988, 285–286), food is not simply a form of physiological sustenance. Our cultural worldviews are reflected in our culinary practices and the way food is classified: what constitutes food, taboos, rules of propriety and conduct, gender and age associations with foods, what is eaten when, food combinations, and whether a food is considered healthful or harmful. His theory of incorporation helps to explain how food customs and identity reflect one another. Put simply, by ingesting a food, one incorporates the properties of the item eaten as it is classified within the cultural system of which one is a part. By doing so, the eater is also seen to be incorporated into the system and the group for which that system has meaning (Fischler 1988, 280–281).

How does this play out in practice? There are clearly foods that speak to us of home and warmth. These are usually the foods of our childhood, items classified as comfort food. The further we are from home, the more meaning these foods have to us – so our food choices can and do reflect our identity. But eating the cuisine of another culture does not necessarily make the eater a member of that culture. We need to ask whether the choice to eat that meal reflects, in part, a choice to ingest the values perceived to be inherent in that meal. When members of a minority culture choose to incorporate foods of the dominant culture, are they choosing to incorporate the values that they see reflected in that food? And if people in the Roman provinces chose what might be labelled Romanized patterns of eating, did that then make them Roman? Were they choosing to incorporate their own perceptions of the values inherent in a so-called Roman diet when doing so? Was something else at play, such as creolization or the incorporation of new items into old layers of meaning (Webster 2001)?

In order to understand how various aspects of identity can be expressed through foodways, I looked at some examples from both the social sciences and examinations of faunal remains from archaeological sites. It would be helpful to take a look at some of the relevant issues they touch upon. Three social science studies in particular stood out: Harbottle's (2000) *Food for Health, Food for Wealth – The Performance of Ethnic and Gender Identities by Iranian Settlers in Britain*, Prasad's (2006) 'Crisis, Identity, and Social Distinction: Cultural Politics of Food, Taste, and Consumption in Late Colonial Bengal', and Wilk's (1999) '"Real Belizean Food": Building Local Identity in the Transnational Caribbean'. The first addresses the expression of ethnic, gender and age-related identity through dietary customs in an immigrant community. The second shows the use of food to express ethnic identity and claim status through the creation of cultural capital within a community in crisis under colonial rule. The third focuses on the use of food to create a national identity in a post-colonial context.

Foodways as a Reflection of Cultural Identity

Some important common denominators emerged in all of these studies: the idea that the foodstuffs of the dominant culture are somehow of a lesser quality than food from home, somehow contaminated, adulterated and unhealthy; that eating these foods is seen to contribute to the contamination of both the physical body and the cultural body of the individual and the group; that even traditional dishes made using ingredients bought from the other are experienced as tasting off, especially by first generation immigrants and those under colonial rule. Conversely, foods from home are idealized as superior and pure, unadulterated, more flavourful and healthier; eating these is seen to counteract the contamination of the physical and cultural body. In order to keep the family physically and culturally healthy, it is important to ensure that children grow up eating these pure, traditional foods. At the same time, in some instances, the value of allowing children some of the foods of their peers was recognized, as a certain amount of assimilation within the dominant culture would be necessary for their upward mobility in society. Harbottle's (2000) work is particularly interesting because it shows how the children of Iranian immigrants absorb the social/psychological conditioning of their families, associating certain foods with home and comfort, while also being able to enjoy aspects of the cuisine of the dominant culture and incorporate them into their culinary vocabulary. This is reflected in their sense of identity, seeing themselves as both British and Iranian.

One of the problems inherent in applying social science models to archaeological scenarios is that archaeologists do not have the benefit of direct contact with members of the groups being studied. Even historical archaeologists are rarely privy to sources that reveal attitudes outside of the dominant culture (see Gray, this volume). Other challenges in trying to bridge the gap between theory and material that we have little or no control over are the distance in time and space between ourselves and the societies we study, and that the material we study is just a fraction of the material that was used. That said, we do have control over other factors: the questions we ask, the designs of our research, and our handling of the material. Material needs to be collected, stored and analysed so that it retains both its contextual and its diachronic meaning. That this is not often done with bone material reflects an attitude that regards faunal remains as secondary to other types of material culture. Faunal remains need to be seen as an asset to interpretation, rather than simply a by-product of excavations.

It seems the most effective attempts to search for identity in the zooarchaeological record are the ones that look at the dietary choices being made by different groups that have access to the same resources. Two that stood out in my research were Ijzereef's (1989) 'Social Differentiation from Animal Bone Studies' and Warner's (2001) 'Ham Hocks on Your Corn Flakes'. Both look at the faunal evidence for food choices being made in various households at a given time and place and compare how different groups were expressing different forms of identity. Ijzereef looked at seventeenth-century cesspits from Jewish and non-Jewish households from the Waterlooplein in Amsterdam and showed how religious, status and cultural identities were visible in dietary choices.

Warner analysed material from a nineteenth-century African-American household in Annapolis, Maryland, and compared it to material from other households in town, both African-American and Anglo-American, showing how the choices being made were a clear reflection of ethnic identity.

For various reasons, expressions of identity come to the fore in periods and places where different groups become inter-dependent. Because of this, expressions of identity should be visible in the Roman frontier province of *Germania Inferior*, especially in areas where military and civilian influences came together. My intention is to test this theory by looking at the faunal remains from the modern town of Nijmegen in the Netherlands, an important strategic site during the Roman occupation that had both a military and civilian presence. Anthony King (1984; 1999) has made important contributions in this area, comparing different types of Roman-period sites, first in Britain and other areas of the north-west provinces, and then across the Empire. King focused on the macro-regional level in order to get a clearer picture of broad trends in dietary identities. My focus will be on a micro-regional level in order to observe different choices made within the same community. My hope is that this will add layers of nuance to what is often a dualistic picture of Roman versus native.

Cultural Identity at Nijmegen

The military presence in Nijmegen during the early Roman period took the form of two camps built around 10 BC, a large offensive base on the Hunerberg and a couple of phases of a smaller command post/cavalry camp on the Kops plateau. A contemporary civilian settlement, thought to be the *Oppidum Batavorum*, was built on the Valkhof starting in the first decade AD (Van Enckevoort *et al.* 2000, 23–40). In the mid-Roman period, after the Batavian revolt of AD 69, the military presence took the form of a large *castra* on the Hunerberg that housed a succession of legions from AD 70–175. Adjacent to this was a *canabae legionis*, a camp village made up of civilians but under the jurisdiction of the commander. A larger civilian presence was the urbanized *Ulpia Noviomagus Batavorum* to the west of the old *Oppidum* containing everything from artisan quarters to bath houses and temples (Van Enckevoort *et al.* 2000, 45–72). By the fourth century, only a small, fortified settlement with associated cemeteries remained (Van Enckevoort *et al.* 2000, 100–105). It has been suggested that this was mainly civilian in nature, but that by this time, all families in the region would have had ties to the military (Willems 1986, 429).

I have examined a number of zooarchaeological reports in order to try to synthesize data for Roman Nijmegen. The contexts represented were six military, five civilian, four mortuary, and two cult complexes. For quantification, I have chosen to look at the Number of Identified Specimens (NISP) as this was the one method common to all the reports. Because a number of reports combined data from multiple features, it was impossible in some cases to determine if bones had come from butchery, kitchen, or consumption waste. Where an assemblage could be identified as butchery waste, it was

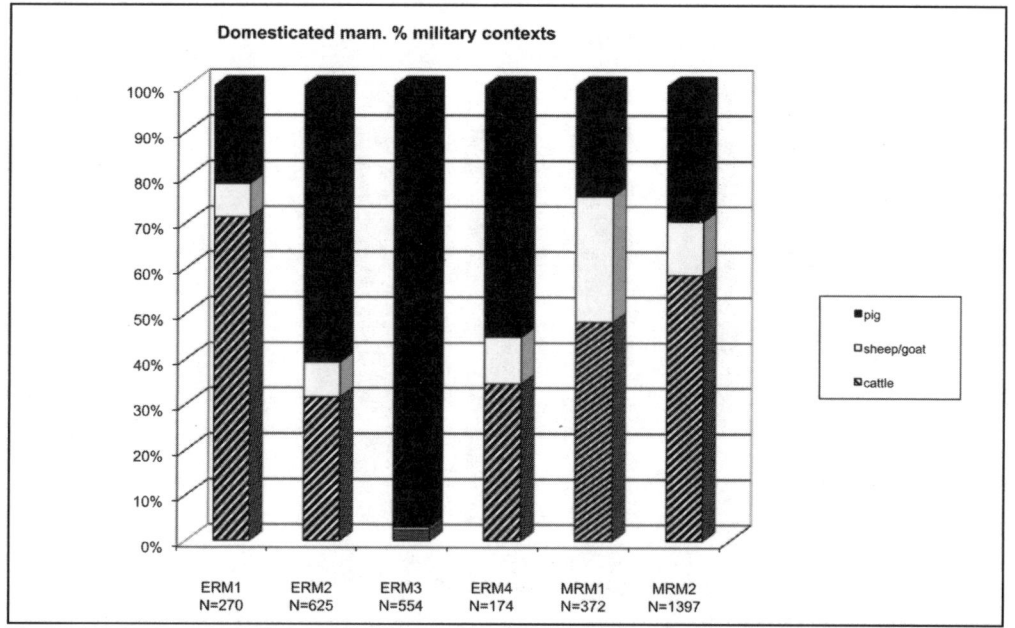

Figure 15.1. Relative percentages of three main domesticates in Early-Roman military (ERM) and Middle Roman military (MRM) contexts in Nijmegen. Contexts from left to right: ERM1 = Valkhof castellum 10 BC–AD 25 (Lauwerier 1988); ERM2 = Hunerberg castra 12 BC–AD 16 (Koopmans 1996); ERM3 = Kops Plateau AD 10–AD 70 (Laarman 1998); ERM4 = Hunerberg castra 'Augustan' (Thijssen 1988); MRM1 = Hunerberg castra AD 70–AD 120 (Thijssen 1988); MRM2 = Hunerberg castra AD 70–AD 120 (Lauwerier 1988).

not included. That some reports may include mixed assemblages should not greatly alter the picture of general species use. In this region, beef seems to have dominated both Iron Age and rural Roman menus, a fact that has been linked to pastoralist ideology (Roymans 1995, 55). Increases in pork and chicken are often seen as Roman influence on indigenous foodways, and I have focused on these species as cultural markers in the assemblages.

Comparing the material from the military and civilian contexts (Figs. 15.1 and 15.2), a pattern emerges. With a couple of notable exceptions, military contexts show more pig and fewer cattle remains than civilian contexts. Looking at averages per period, cattle percentages in military contexts increase through time from 35 to 53 per cent, while pig decreases from 58 to 27 per cent. In civilian contexts, pig representation is low (between 15 and 20 per cent) through three centuries, while cattle remains dominate, ranging from 64 to 84 per cent.

The picture that emerges suggests a consistency in civilian assemblages that may point to cultural continuity in local foodways. At the same time, even though beef consumption in military contexts never comes close to approximating that in civilian

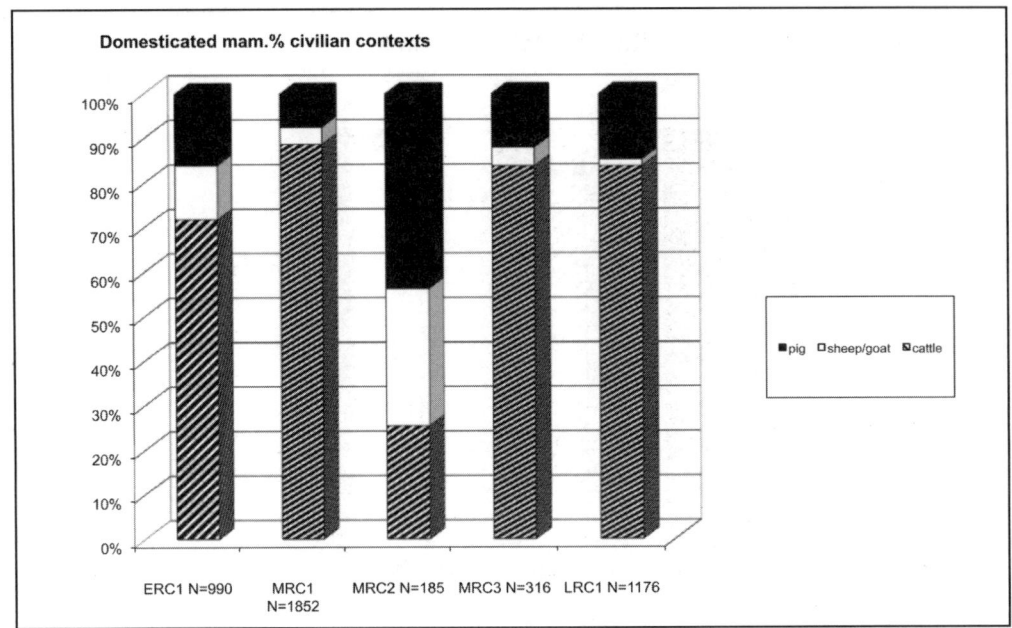

Figure 15.2. Relative percentages of three main domesticates in civilian contexts in Nijmegen. Contexts from left to right: Early-Roman civilian (ERC1) = Oppidum Batavorum AD 40– AD 70 (Lauwerier 1988); Mid-Roman civilian 1 (MRC1) = Hunerberg canabae AD 70– AD 120 (ibid.); Mid-Roman civilian 2 (MRC2) = Hunerberg canabae AD 70–AD 120 (Koopmans 1996); Mid-Roman civilian 3 (MRC3) = Hunerberg canabae AD 70–AD 90 (Rijkelijkhuizen 2001); LRC1 = Valkhof settlement AD 330–AD 350 (Lauwerier 1988).

contexts, the increase in beef within army sites might indicate a creolization, mixing local food cultures with those from abroad.

Another possibility for glimpsing cultural reflections in foodways is provided by non-daily food customs, such as cult offerings and burial meals. It can be argued that the identities expressed in these contexts are public identities, reflecting how people wanted to be seen, rather than the private identities expressed in daily diet. I looked at two cult complexes, the early/mid-Roman temple at Elst, thought to be dedicated to the indigenous deity Hercules Magusanus (Roymans 2004, 242), and the mid-Roman Fortuna temple in Nijmegen, dedicated to the Roman goddess Fortuna (Fig. 15.3). For both periods at Elst, cattle comprises 93 per cent of the assemblage. At the Fortuna Temple, where cattle are absent, chicken accounts for 97 per cent of the material. Unlike the ambiguousness of daily food choices, here the relevance of species as cultural markers becomes clear.

Similarly, in mortuary contexts, public identities seem to take precedence. I looked at the early/mid-Roman Nijmegen Hatert cemetery, and the late-Roman Margriet and Binnenstad cemeteries. Although poor preservation means that the data from these

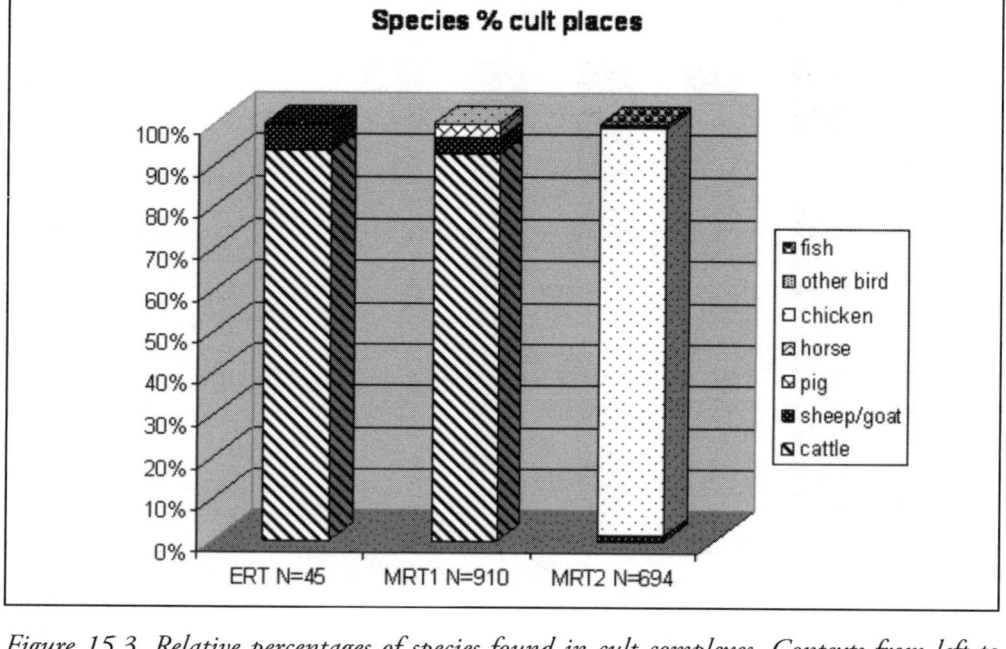

Figure 15.3. Relative percentages of species found in cult complexes. Contexts from left to right: Early-Roman Temple 1 (ERT1) = Elst, pre-temple phase, ??BC–AD 50 (Lauwerier 1988); Mid-Roman Temple 1 (MRT1) = Elst, Temple Period AD 50–3rd century (ibid.); Mid-Roman Temple 2 (MRT2) = Fortuna Temple 2nd century AD (Zeiler 1997).

contexts cannot be used for quantitative analysis, they remain qualitatively valuable. In contrast to the associated Valkhof settlement, beef seems to be almost absent from the graves, but this could be due to the use of fillets. What is most intriguing, however, is the dominance of pig and chicken in graves especially when compared to the associated settlement where chicken is practically absent.

Conclusion

The pattern that seems to emerge regarding daily dietary choices would indicate a large degree of continuity in local food cultures despite the imperial presence. The increase in beef and decrease in pork through time in the military contexts may even indicate that local foodways had a greater influence on the military diet than the other way around. The huge disparities in assemblages from cult complexes may result from the ideological ordering of species within cultural worldviews, while the dominance of pork and chicken in graves in contrast to their associated settlement may illustrate differences in public and private forms of identity.

To conclude, I would like to return to some of my earlier points. It seems that given the chance, the social sciences are well equipped to provide archaeologists with a theoretical vocabulary regarding identity. Because identity can be reflected in food habits, foodways can provide us with a window through which identity can be viewed. I believe that this reflection is visible in the zooarchaeological record and that it is possible, as exemplified by the Nijmegen case study, to glimpse how identities were expressed on a micro-level in the Roman provinces.

References

Diaz-Andreu, M., S. Lucy, S. Babic and Edwards, D. N. 2005. *The Archaeology of Identity: Approaches to Gender, Age, Status, Ethnicity and Religion* (London).

Fischler, C. 1988. 'Food, self and identity', *Social Science Information* **27** (2), 275–292.

Harbottle, L. 2000. *Food for Health, Food for Wealth: The Performance of Ethnic and Gender Identities by Iranian Settlers in Britain* (New York).

Ijzereef, G. E. 1989. 'Social differentiation from animal bone studies', in Serjeantson, D. and Waldron, T. (eds) *Diet and Crafts in Towns: The Evidence of Animal Remains from the Roman to the Post-Medieval Periods* (Oxford), 41–53.

Jones, S. 1997. *The Archaeology of Ethnicity: Constructing Identities in the Past and Present* (London).

King, A. 1984. 'Animal bones and the dietary identity of military and civilian groups in Roman Britain, Germany and Gaul', in Blagg, T. F. C. and King, A. C. (eds) *Military and Civilian in Roman Britain: Cultural Relationships in a Frontier Province* (Oxford), 187–217.

King, A. 1999. 'Diet in the Roman world: a regional inter-site comparison of the mammal bones', *Journal of Roman Archaeology* **12**, 168–202.

Koopmans, L. 1996. *Vroeg-Romeins botmateriaal van de Hunerberg te Nijmegen* Unpublished PhD thesis, University of Amsterdam.

Laarman, F. J. 1998. *Nijmegen Kops Plateau: Het Botmateriaal uit Twee Vroeg-Romeinse Latrines. Internal Report Archaeozoology* (Amersfoort).

Lauwerier, R. C. G. M. 1988. *Animals in Roman Times in the Dutch Eastern River Area*, Neaderrlandse Oudheden 12, ROB (Amersfoort).

Prasad, S. 2006. 'Crisis, identity, and social distinction: cultural politics of food, taste, and consumption in late colonial Bengal', *Journal of Historical Sociology* **19** (3), 245–265.

Rijkelijkhuizen, M. 2001. *Dierlijke resten in Romeins Nijmegen*. PhD thesis, University of Amsterdam.

Roymans, N. 1995. 'Romanization, cultural identity and the ethnic discussion: the integration of Lower Rhine populations in the Roman Empire', in Metzler, J., Millet, M., Roymans, N. and Slofstra, J. (eds) *Integration in the Early Roman West: The Role of Culture and Ideology*. (Luxembourg), 47–64.

Roymans, N. 2004. *Ethnic Identity and Imperial Power: The Batavians in the Early Roman Empire* (Amsterdam).

Thijssen, J. R. A. M. 1988. *Romeins Botmateriaal uit Nijmegen en Woerden*. Unpublished PhD thesis, University of Amsterdam.

Van Enckevoort, H., Haalebos, J. K. and Thijssen, J. 2000. *Nijmegen: Legerplaats en stad in het Achterland van de Romeinse Limes* (Abcoude).

Warner, M. 2001. 'Ham Hocks on Your Cornflakes', *Archaeology* **54** (6), 48–52.

Webster, J. 2001. 'Creolizing the Roman Provinces', *American Journal of Archaeology* **105** (2), 209–225.

Wilk, R. R. 1999. '"Real Belizean Food": building local identity in the transnational Caribbean', *American Anthropologist* **101** (2), 244–255.

Willems, J. H. W. 1986. *Romans and Batavians: a Regional Study in the Dutch Eastern River Area*. Unpublished PhD thesis, University of Amsterdam.

Zeiler, J. T. 1997. 'Offers en slachtoffers: faunaresten uit de Fortunatempel te Nijmegen (2^e eeuw n.Chr.)' *Paleo-Aktueel* **8**, 105–107.

Website 1: 'Identity', The American Heritage® Dictionary of the English Language. Houghton Mifflin Company. Fourth Edition, Online http://dictionary.reference.com/browse/identity. Accessed 03 Nov. 2006.

The Pewsey Middens:
Centres of Feasting or Symbols of Community?

Andy Tullett, University of Leicester
and
Chris Harrison, University of Sheffield

Introduction

Over the last 25 years, research within and around the Vale of Pewsey (Wiltshire) has unearthed evidence suggesting that the area was the centre of Late Bronze Age/Earliest Iron Age activity. Eight potential midden sites have been identified, with investigations focusing on those at Potterne (Lawson 2000) and East Chisenbury (McOmish 1996). More recently, between 2003 and 2004, the University of Sheffield led a programme of research to re-assess the All Cannings Cross midden and investigate a new site at Stanton St Bernard. All these sites are characterized by thick (1.5–2.0m) deposits of dark humic material rich in animal bone, ceramics and artefacts, seemingly laid down over relatively short periods, perhaps as little as 100 years (David Field pers. comm.).

McOmish (1996, 75) links the appearance of these middens to broad changes in the symbols of society, such as a new emphasis on boundaries, with the creation of the linear earthwork systems, and a shift from open to enclosed settlement. These are taken as indicators of an increasingly competitive society with the middens representing the remains of 'ceremonial feasting places'. It has been suggested that feasting occasions were socially divisive, the élite utilizing agricultural surplus to negotiate status, influence and wealth, and to create reciprocal obligations upon which they might draw in the future (Barrett *et al.* 1991). This paper seeks to offer an alternative perspective on the physical and psychological function of the Pewsey middens. It focuses on recent work at All Cannings Cross, Stanton St Bernard and, where pertinent, draws upon the Potterne and East Chisenbury material. By integrating the landscape evidence with that from animal remains and contemporary trends in material culture, it is suggested that the midden sites were a focus for disparate groups and, rather than being socially divisive, may actually have been symbols of community.

Landscape Setting

The Vale of Pewsey in Wiltshire is situated between the Marlborough Downs to the north and Salisbury Plain to the south. It is approximately 20km long by 5km wide and its steep chalk scarps are littered with monuments dating from the Neolithic to the Iron Age. During the Late Bronze and Early Iron Age, a large system of linear earthworks was laid out across the downs, in some cases running across earlier Middle Bronze Age field systems that were apparently abandoned at this time (Gingell 1992, 158). This dramatic reorganization of the landscape, which has been linked to an increasing emphasis on pastoralism as well as territorial or tenurial divisions (McOmish *et al.* 2002, 64; Cunliffe 2004), must have affected how the area was utilized, traversed and perceived. For instance, the linear earthworks, rather than acting simply as barriers (as suggested by Cunliffe 2004, 74), probably facilitated the structured movement of humans and their livestock by creating direct routes across long distances where the intricacies of the Middle Bronze Age field systems had previously impeded passage (Hawkes 1939, 147). The possibility that linear earthwork systems played a role as routes or droveways is indicated by the example at Dunch Hill where a hollow-way parallels the line of a linear earthwork (Bradley *et al.* 1994, 128).

Towards the end of the Late Bronze Age, early hilltop enclosures were created at nodal points in the system. For instance, at Martinsell, itself the site of a potential midden, an enclosure was laid out with a linear earthwork forming its northern boundary (Cunliffe 2004, 72), whilst the East Chisenbury midden was deposited within an enclosure that is the focus of six linear earthworks (McOmish *et al.* 2002, 58). Early hilltop enclosures rarely show much settlement activity and the fact that they are so closely associated with the linear earthwork systems suggests that both were part of an integrated system of stock management, the hilltop enclosures used to corral animals for shearing, lambing or division between the owners (Cunliffe 2004, 75). Rybury Hillfort, which overlooks the sites of All Cannings Cross and Stanton St Bernard appears to have been an early hilltop enclosure but it has been largely destroyed by historic quarrying, so preventing its investigation. In summary, in the period immediately prior to the formation of the middens, it seems that the landscape was being re-organized on a large scale to facilitate new animal management strategies. The possibility that these landscape changes were accompanied by wider shifts in material culture will now be considered.

Ceramics

The standard ceramic assemblage for Late Bronze Age Wessex is Post Deverel-Rimbury 'Plain' ware, which consists of sparsely decorated, straight-walled vessel types. By the Earliest Iron Age these forms were replaced by All Cannings Cross wares. The change is quite dramatic in both style and vessel forms: bowls and cups appear and all ceramic forms have a much greater degree of decoration. The fine wares, such as furrowed and scratched cordoned bowls, are a complete contrast to earlier fine wares; however such vessels are found on all types of Early Iron Age site, suggesting that they were freely available and not restricted to any single social stratum (Morris 1996, 43). Whilst it is accepted that bowls and cups may have existed in organic forms prior to the Earliest Iron Age (Barrett 1980b, 313) the developments in form and decoration are usually considered to be synchronous with an increase in emphasis on the preparation and service of food.

The Pewsey Middens

In most respects the Pewsey midden ceramics are consistent with the standard assemblages of the Earliest Iron Age. There is, however, one area in which they differ considerably: the middens contain a noticeable presence of vessels with perforated bases that, elsewhere, are rare until the Late Iron Age (Gingell and Morris 2000, 153). It is thought that these vessels acted as strainers and relate to a specialized aspect of food processing (Gingell and Morris 2000, 153), perhaps straining the curd for cheese production. To investigate this possibility further we will test this hypothesis against a study of the animal bone data to which we now turn.

Faunal remains

All of the Pewsey middens excavated to date have yielded exceptionally large quantities of animal bone. For the East Chisenbury assemblage it has been estimated that over 3,800 caprines, 600 cattle and 450 pigs must have been slaughtered annually to account for the faunal remains represented at the site (Serjeantson *et al.* forthcoming). The meat from these animals would have been sufficient to have fed a resident population of between 750 (Bagust 1996, 67) and 2000 (Serjeantson *et al.* forthcoming) over the 100 years of its existence.

The animal remains from All Cannings Cross and Stanton St Bernard are displayed in table 16.1. As with most sites across the United Kingdom, they are dominated by domesticates (Grant 1984; Hambleton 1999) and, in common with other sites in Wessex, the assemblages contain high frequencies of caprine remains (Grant 1984 and 1991; Hambleton 1999; Cunliffe 2004). It should be noted that, although sheep/goats dominate all the Vale of Pewsey midden sites, cattle would have been the main source of meat due to their larger carcass size (Bagust 1996, 67).

The sheep/goat mortality profile for All Cannings Cross and Stanton St Bernard is displayed in table 16.2. From this it is clear that there was a peak in mortalities between six and twelve months. Hambleton (1999) has suggested that yearling sheep would have been slaughtered towards the end of autumn after grazing on the stubble of fields but before winter conditions prevailed. Figure 16.1 shows the Stanton St Bernard cull-pattern compared to profiles from two contemporary sites: Danebury, where a milk/meat economy has been suggested (Grant 1984, 511–2) and West Cotton, where wool was deemed to be the dominant product (Albarella and Davis 1994). It can be seen that the Stanton St Bernard profile shares many more similarities with that of Danebury than West Cotton, suggesting that sheep/goats from this site were being exploited as part of a meat and dairy regime. This is interesting given that recent analysis of animal lipids from prehistoric pottery, including sherds from the nearby midden at Potterne, has highlighted the importance of processed dairy products in this period: of the Potterne vessels containing lipids, 60 per cent related to ruminant dairy fats (Copley *et al.* 2005).

Several possible conclusions may be drawn from the All Cannings Cross and Stanton St Bernard faunal remains. The first is that cattle, although slaughtered in lower

	ALL CANNINGS CROSS						STANTON ST BERNARD							
	In situ		Topsoil/Ploughsoil		Total		In situ		Derived		Ploughsoil		Total	
	n	%	n	%	n	%	n	%	n	%	n	%	n	%
Cattle	50	22%	55	27%	105	25%	78	21%	14	15%	3	17%	95	20%
Sheep/goat	158	70%	119	59%	277	65%	241	65%	62	67%	10	56%	313	65%
Sheep	2		7		9		58		12		1		69	
Goat	0		0		0		10		1		0		11	
Pig	10	4%	19	9%	29	7%	50	14%	15	18%	2	11%	67	14%
Equid	4	2%	6	3%	10	2%	1	0%	2	2%	3	17%	6	1%
Red deer	0	0%	0 (+1)	0%	0 (+1)	0%	0	0%	0	0%	0	0%	0	0%
Roe deer	1	0%	0	0%	1	0%	0	0%	0	0%	0	0%	0	0%
Dog	2	1%	1	0%	3	1%	0	0%	0	0%	0	0%	0	0%
Rat	0	0%	1	0%	1	0%	0	0%	0	0%	0	0%	0	0%
Total	225		201		426		370		93		18		481	

Table 16.1. Numbers of mammal bones (NISP) All Cannings Cross and Stanton St Bernard. All levels are represented. 'Non-countable' evidence used to denote the presence of a species are noted as + and then a number. Sheep/goat includes the specimens identified to species. Pig and ruminant half distal metapodials have been divided by two. All equid incisors have been divided by two due to the difficulty of differentiating mandibular and maxillary specimens.

Wear stage	Sheep/goat	Sheep	Goat	%
A				0
B	5	4	1	25
C	6	5	1	30
D	2	2		10
E	1	1		5
F	2			10
G	1			5
H	1			5
I	2			10
Total	20	12	2	100

Table 16.2. Mandibular wear stages in sheep from Stanton St Bernard. Mandibles with two or more teeth (with recordable wear stage) are displayed. The wear stages follow Payne (1973): A=0–2m, B=2–6m, C=6–12m, D+1–2y, E=2–3y, F=3–4y, G=4–6y, H=6–8y, I=8–10y (m=months, y=years).

numbers than sheep/goats, were still the most important source of meat at the middens. Second, caprines appear to have been managed for both meat and dairy products. Third, there appears to be a significant degree of seasonality in the slaughter patterns.

Competition or Community?

It is now apparent that the Pewsey middens were a phenomenon of the Earliest Iron Age, established soon after the construction of the linear earthwork systems on the surrounding downs. The linear earthwork systems and early hilltop enclosures both point to the increasing importance of pastoralism at this time. The ceramic forms and styles of All Cannings Cross wares indicate the preparation and service of food, whilst the decorative nature of these vessels suggests that display during consumption was of particular importance. The presence of strainers at the middens, when they are rare on other types of site, indicates that some form of specialized food production was limited to these locations. When considered in conjunction with lipid analysis and the sheep/goat mortality profiles, processed dairy fats, such as cheese, seem the most likely product. The large quantity of faunal remains, in particular from East Chisenbury, suggests that considerable numbers of animals, derived from substantial herds, were being slaughtered annually. Whilst this in turn suggests that these sites could sustain large permanent populations, the seasonality in the sheep/goat mortality profiles hints that human presence at the sites may have fluctuated through the year.

At first glimpse, none of this appears to contradict current interpretations of the sites as occasional centres of competitive feasting; however, there are other facts that make

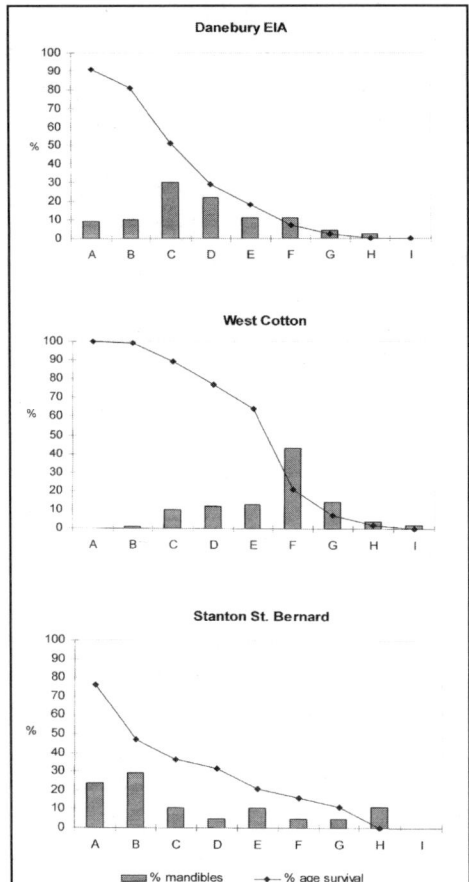

Figure 16.1. Sheep mortality at Stanton St Bernard compared to Early Iron Age (EIA) Danebury and Iron Age West Cotton.

this scenario more difficult to uphold. For instance, Brück (2000, 275–6) has argued that concepts of prehistoric people maximizing economic output to meet social aims are problematic. Indeed, it appears that foremost to most subsistence farmers is the minimization of risk, rather than the maximization of output (Netting 1974, 44). It is also clear from studies of the region that the Earliest Iron Age was a period of comparative egalitarianism (Collis 1996, 91). This idea is supported by the faunal remains: the sheer numbers of animals represented suggests that we are looking at communal herds rather than flocks belonging to individual households (Cunliffe 2004, 74).

It is also pertinent to note that one of the main characteristics of the Pewsey middens is the dark earth component that forms the majority of the deposits. Micromorphological and microchemical investigation of this soil at Potterne and East Chisenbury suggest that it consists primarily of burnt and partially decomposed herbivore stabling residues (Macphail 2000, 70; forthcoming). This indicates that the dominant activity taking place at middens was animal management rather than feasting. True, if these sites were centres of competitive feasting we would expect a short-lived influx of animals but evidence suggests that livestock were corralled and stabled in the area for considerable periods of time. Indeed, Serjeantson (2007, 89) has suggested that the build up of byre material reflects an intensive animal management programme whereby animals were brought into the settlement area for milking. Certainly the animal bone assemblage suggests that a dairying element was present at Stanton St Bernard and similar patterns may be identified at Potterne and East Chisenbury. That said, the seasonality of the sheep/goat assemblage indicates that, for the majority of the year, the large caprine herds were managed away from the valley, perhaps on the rougher pasture of the downs.

Division of the animals would have involved division of the community, with different activity groups separated for periods of the year. Such activity groups tend to be drawn along age and gender lines (Chadwick 2007), implying a dramatic fragmentation of these communities. However, the demands of herd management at particular times of the year, such as at lambing or fleecing, would have required a concentration of the community's labour force, bringing these disparate groups back together again. For Stanton St Bernard and All Cannings Cross such activities may have been conducted at the nearby Rybury enclosure.

The separation of these activity groups during the year could lead to tensions upon their return. It would therefore be of paramount importance to find a means of negotiating their re-entry into the community. Fundamental to this could have been the preparation and service of food, utilizing the new ceramic forms of the All Cannings Cross wares and the use of etiquette to structure behaviour. Indeed, we propose that food and its service were used as a means of mediating these reunions and reconstituting the social bonds between groups within the community. Sharing food and drink was however only the vehicle of integration, as it was the interaction during and after the meals that would recreate the social links. It provided the opportunity to share news, stories and jokes, strengthening the links between people. As such, to the people visiting these sites, they may have become symbolically entwined with the identity of community, representing the agricultural cycle, old friends and a series of arrivals and departures.

Conclusion

The middens situated within the Vale of Pewsey are truly remarkable sites. Substantial amounts of material reflecting consumption have been recovered from the middens but these have attracted more attention than the major anthropogenic deposit of the soil. Current accounts reflect this bias and are dominated by discussions of competitive feasting, whereby individuals jostled for power through the manipulation of agricultural surpluses. These arguments outline interactions similar to those proposed for gift exchange with an authority/obligation relationship between the two parties (Barrett 1989, 307). Considering the sites solely in these terms restricts the range of social inquiry to the level of meta-narratives of subordinate/insubordinate relationships.

It therefore prevents a more nuanced understanding of the complex web of social interaction between the people that visited these sites.

We feel that a richer narrative can be created by viewing these sites as gateways between two different but complementary agricultural regimes and sub-communal activity groups. When considered from this perspective it is possible to explore the interactions between sections of community without reverting to traditional discourse based on status and power. Instead of representing a highly competitive and divisive system of social manipulation we may start to see the midden sites as symbolically entwined with the concept of community and co-operation.

References

Albarella U. and Davis S. 1994. *The Saxon and Medieval Animal Bones Excavated 1985–1989 from West Cotton, Northamptonshire*. Unpublished AML report 17/94, English Heritage.

Bagust, J. 1996. *The Animal Bones from Easy Chisenbury, Wiltshire: Ritual Rubbish or Simply a Midden Deposit*. Unpublished MA Dissertation, University of Leicester.

Barrett, J. C., Bradley, R. and Green, M. 1991. *Landscape, Monuments and Society: The Prehistory of Cranbourne Chase* (Cambridge).

Barrett, J. C. 1980a. 'The evolution of Later Bronze Age Settlement', In Barrett, J. C. and Bradley, R. (eds) *Settlement and Society in the British Later Bronze Age* (Oxford), 77–100.

Barrett, J. C. 1980b. 'The pottery of the Later Bronze Age in lowland England', *Proceedings of the Prehistoric Society* **46**, 297–319.

Barrett, J. C. 1989. 'Food, Gender and metal: questions of social reproduction'. In M. L. S. Sorensen and R. Thomas (eds) *The Bronze Age – Iron Age Transition in Europe* (Oxford), 304–320.

Bradley, R., Entwistle, R. and Raymond, F. 1994. *Prehistoric Land Divisions on Salisbury Plain: The Work of the Wessex Linear Ditches Project* (London).

Brück, J. 2000. 'Settlement, landscape and social identity: the Early-Middle Bronze Age transition in Wessex, Sussex and the Thames Valley', *Oxford Journal of Archaeology* **19** (3), 273–300.

Chadwick, A. M. 2007. 'Trackways, hooves and memory days: human and animal movements and memories around the Iron Age and Romano-British rural landscapes of the English North Midlands', in Cummings, V. and Johnston, R. (eds) *Prehistoric Journeys* (Oxford).

Collis, J. R. 1996. 'Hill-forts, enclosures and boundaries', in Champion, T. C. and Collis, J. R. (eds) *The Iron Age in Britain and Ireland: Recent Trends* (Sheffield), 87–94.

Copley, M. S., Berstan, R., Dudd, S. N., Aillaud, S., Mukherjee, A. J., Straker, V., Payne, S. and Evershed, R. P. 2005. 'Processing of milk products in pottery vessels through British prehistory', *Antiquity* **79**, 895–908.

Cunliffe, B. 2004. 'Wessex cowboys?', *Oxford Journal of Archaeology* **23** (1), 61–81.

Dietler, M. 1996. 'Feasts and commensal politics in the political economy: food, power and status in Prehistoric Europe', in Wiessner, P. and Schiefenhövel, W. (eds) *Food and the Status Quest: An Interdisciplinary Perspective* (Berghahn), 87–125.

Gingell, C. 1992. *The Marlborough Downs: A Later Bronze Age Landscape and its Origins* (Devizes).

Gingell, C. J. and Morris, E. L. 2000. 'Form series, section 6 – the artefacts', in Lawson, A. J. (ed.) *Potterne 1982–5: Animal Husbandry in Later Prehistoric Wiltshire* (Salisbury), 149–53.

Grant, A. 1984. 'Animal husbandry in Wessex and the Thames Valley', in Cunliffe, B. and Miles, D. (eds) *Aspects of the Iron Age in Central Southern Britain* (Oxford), 102–119.

Grant, A. 1991. 'Economic or symbolic? Animals and ritual behaviour', in Garwood, P., Jennings, D.,

Skeates R. and Toms, J. (eds) *Sacred and Profane: Proceedings of a Conference on Archaeology, Ritual and Religion. Oxford 1989* (Oxford),109–114.

Hambleton, E., 1999. *Animal Husbandry Regimes in Iron Age Britain: A Comparative Study of Faunal Assemblages from British Iron Age Sites* (Oxford).

Hawkes, C. F. C. 1939. 'The excavations at Quarley Hill, 1938', *Papers and Proceedings of the Hampshire Field Club and Archaeological Society* **14** (2), 136–194.

Jones, M. 2002. 'Eating for calories or company? Concluding remarks on consuming passions', in Miracle, P. and Milner, N. (eds) *Consuming Passions and Patterns of Consumption* (Oxford), 131–136.

Lawson, A. J. 2000. *Potterne 1982–5: Animal Husbandry in Later Prehistoric Wiltshire* (Salisbury).

Macphail, R. I. 2000. 'Soils and microstratigraphy: a soil micromorphological and microchemical approach', in Lawson, A. J. (ed.) *Potterne 1982–5: Animal Husbandry in Later Prehistoric Wiltshire* (Salisbury), 47–71.

Macphail, R. I. Forthcoming. 'A brief assessment of the soil micromorphoology', in Brown, G. Field, D. and McOmish, D. *The Late Bronze Age – Early Iron Age Site at East Chisenbury, Wiltshire*.

McOmish, D., Field, D. and Brown, G. 2002. *The Field Archaeology of the Salisbury Plain Training Area* (Swindon).

McOmish, D. 1996. 'East Chisenbury: ritual and rubbish at the British Bronze Age – Iron Age transition', *Antiquity* **70**, 68–76.

Morris, E. L. 1996. 'Iron Age artefact production and exchange', in Champion, T. C. and Collis, J. R. (eds) *The Iron Age in Britain and Ireland: Recent Trends* (Sheffield), 41–65.

Netting, R. M. 1974. 'Agrarian ecology', *Annual Review of Anthropology* **3**, 21–56.

Payne, S. 1973. 'Kill-off patterns in sheep and goats: the mandibles from Asvan Kale', *Anatolian Studies* **23**, 281–303.

Rowlands, M. J. 1980. 'Kinship, alliance and exchange in the European Bronze Age', in Barrett, J. C. and Bradley, R. (eds) *The British Later Bronze Age* (Oxford), 15–55.

Serjeantson, D. 2007. 'Intensification of animal husbandry in the Late Bronze Age?', in Haselgrove C. and Pope, R. (eds) *The Earlier Iron Age in Britain and the Near Continent* (Oxford), 80–93.

Serjeantson, D., Bagust, J. and Jenkins, C. forthcoming. 'Animal Bone', in Brown, G., Field, D. and McOmish, D. *The Late Bronze Age – Early Iron Age Site at East Chisenbury, Wiltshire*.

	Herdonia (4th–first half of 5th c.)			Herdonia (end of 5th–7th c.)			Faragola (second half of 6th c.)				Canosa, San Pietro (end of 6th–7th c.)			
	NISP	%	MNI	NISP	%	MNI	NISP	%	MNI	%	NISP	%	MNI	%
Cattle	375	34.6	36	947	46.6	74	139	33	14	21.8	20	11.4	6	21.4
Sheep/goats	426	41.2	50	625	32.7	80	183	49	18	46.8	67	39.6	8	35.7
Sheep	6			25		9	15		6		2		2	
Goats	14			15		4	10		6					
Pigs	216	19.9	48	387	19	69	65	15.2	14	21.8	58	33.3	8	28.5
Fowl	45	4.1	19	29	1.4	25	14	3.2	6	9.3	27	15.5	4	14.2
Total ID	1082		153	2028		261	426		64		174		28	

Table 17.1. *Number of Identified Specimens (NISP) and Minimum Number of Individuals (MNI) of the principal domestic animals from fourth to sixth/seventh centuries.*

	Herdonia (7th–10th c.)			Faragola (end of 6th–7th/8th c.)			Canosa, San Pietro (end of 7th–8th c.)				Canosa, San Pietro (9th–10th c.)			
	NISP	%	MNI	NISP	%	MNI	NISP	%	MNI	%	NISP	%	MNI	%
Cattle	590	35.7	56	104	17.5	15	99	9	17	12.9	183	9.23	26	9.3
Sheep/goats	615	40.3	50	261	47.5	31	455	43.2	32	29	1023	51.8	113	42.2
Sheep	30		10	12		5	5		2		3		2	
Goats	21		8	9		5	12		4		5		2	
Pigs	238	14.4	53	143	24.1	43	401	36.7	54	41.2	409	20.6	61	22
Fowl	157	9.5	23	64	10.7	16	119	10.9	22	16.7	359	18.1	73	26.3
Total ID	1651		200	593		115	1091		131		1982		277	

Table 17.2. *Number of Identified Specimens (NISP) and Minimum Number of Individuals (MNI) of the principal domestic animals from seventh to tenth centuries.*

Zooarchaeological Research in Apulia, Southern Italy: Some Considerations of Animal Exploitation from Late Antiquity to the Early Middle Ages

Antonietta Buglione,
University of Foggia

Introduction

This work represents part of a broader archaeological project led by Prof. G. Volpe (University of Foggia, Italy) on the Roman and medieval settlements of northern Apulia (Southern Italy). The zooarchaeological research focuses on the period between Late Antiquity to the Early Middle Ages, *ca.* fifth to tenth century AD. It aims to reconstruct aspects of the production and consumption of animals in relation to people and the environment.

The animal bone samples considered within this paper come from the Roman city of Herdonia, the San Pietro Hill at Canosa di Puglia and the Roman villa of Faragola at Ascoli Satriano (Tables 17.1 and 17.2). They have been examined using the methods of Buglione (2006).

Materials

Tables 17.1 and 17.2 show the composition of the assemblages from the different sites and periods. The data are shown in terms of both the Number of Identified Specimens (NISP) and the Minimum Number of Individuals (MNI).

At Herdonia, pigs and sheep/goats were the most exploited animals during the Roman period (second to third centuries), bred and slaughtered locally; whereas wild animal remains are few (Leguilloux 2000, 478–481). In the fourth to fifth centuries, sheep and goats became the most abundant taxon according to both the NISP and MNI, followed by cattle and pigs. Sheep/goats were bred for wool and dairy products, in addition to meat. Pigs were killed at every age, with sucking pigs making up 34 per cent of the ageable sample (n = 47). Cattle were more frequently slaughtered after four or five years of age, when they were no longer agriculturally useful. During the late fifth to seventh centuries, Herdonia suffered a phase of reduction and instability. At this time ,meat from pigs became an important product, probably due to its low production costs, and 49 per cent of individuals (n = 47) were killed between two to three years of age. Cattle remains also became more numerous than in previous centuries and most derive from animals used in field activities.

The bone samples collected from the ruin layers of the Roman villa at Faragola (Volpe *et al.* 2005) and the Late Antique ecclesiastic complex at Canosa di Puglia, San Pietro Hill (Volpe *et al.* 2007) confirm that pastoral use of sheep and goats for wool, milk and meat was widespread in the late sixth/seventh centuries (Table 17.1). Whereas at Herdonia sheep/goats were killed to obtain wool and meat, the ageing data for seventh- to eighth-century San Pietro village indicate a greater emphasis on milk production. Besides the local breeding and consumption of domestic animals at Herdonia, San Pietro and Faragola, skeletal representation data indicate that animals and their body parts were probably exchanged and traded.

Domestic bird remains from Herdonia, San Pietro and Faragola suggest that both poultry and eggs were important alimentary resources. An increase in poultry between the seventh and tenth centuries may reflect major developments in medieval bird breeding which occurred as their value as providers of meat and eggs became widely recognized (Benecke 1993, 24–28).

The remains of wild animals (deer, wild boar and hare) are represented in low frequencies at all sites, suggesting that they did not contribute significantly to the diet, instead being regarded as occasional food resource. Based on the remains, it is not possible to determine if their low frequency indicates a limited presence of woodland in the settlements' hinterland or limited access to woodland in general.

From the seventh century onwards, fish and shellfish increased as a food source, particularly at Faragola and San Pietro. This suggests that at least some trade was taking place between the coast and inland sites. Some of the oyster shells exhibit holes on their valves. It is possible that these holes were created by natural predators or were caused by breeding techniques in oyster beds. More probable is Reese's (2002) suggestion that the shells were pierced so that they might be linked together and packed in ice or snow for transport.

Conclusion

From the fourth to tenth centuries, the animal economy of Apulia was founded on exploitation of domesticates that satisfied the rural population's demands for primary (meat) and secondary (milk and wool) products. The zooarchaeological data suggest that sheep/goats were the most important resource in northern Apulia throughout the period under consideration. Such large-scale caprine husbandry would probably have required extensive pastures and possibly also necessitated transhumance. Wild animals were seemingly of less economic importance, although some trade in fish and shellfish is indicated.

Acknowledgments

Thanks to Prof. G. Volpe for letting me to begin these zooarchaeological researches and continuing to offer assistance; thanks to C. Minniti and Prof. J. De Grossi Mazzorin for help in different stages of the research. Thanks to N. Sykes for accepting my paper and for having read and corrected it.

References

Benecke, N. 1993. 'On the use of the domestic fowl in the Central Europe from the Iron Age to the Middle Age', *Archeofauna* 2, 21–31.

Buglione, A. 2006. 'Ricerche archeozoologiche in Puglia centro-settentrionale: primi dati sullo sfruttamnto della risorsa animale fra Tardoantico e Altomedioevo', in Gravina A. (ed.) *Atti del 26° Convegno sulla Preistoria, Protostoria e Storia della Daunia, San Severo 2005* (San Severo), 495–532.

Leguilloux, M. 2000. 'Le matériel ostéologique d'Ordona. Campagnes de fouilles 194–1995 : premières conclusions', in Volpe G. (ed.) *Ordona X. Ricerche archeologiche ad Herdonia (1993–1998)* (Bari), 477–496.

Reese, D. S. 2002. 'Marine and fresh-water shells', in Mackinnon M. R. (ed.) *The Excavations of San Giovanni di Ruoti: The Faunal and Plant Remains* (London), 189–193.

Volpe, G., De Felice G., Turchiano M. 2005. 'Faragola (Ascoli Satriano): Una residenza aristocratica tardoantica e un villaggio altomedievale nella Valle del Carapelle: primi dati', in Volpe G., Turchiano M. (eds) *Paesaggi e Insediamenti Rurali in Italia Meridionale fra Tardoantico e Altomedioevo* (Bari), 265–298.

Volpe, G., Favia, P., Giuliani, R., Nuzzo, D. 2007. 'Il complesso sabiniano di S. Pietro a Canosa', in Bonacasa Carra M., Vitale M. (eds) *La Cristianizzazione in Italia fra Tardoantico e Altomedieovo: Aspetti e Problemi* (Palermo), 1113–1165.

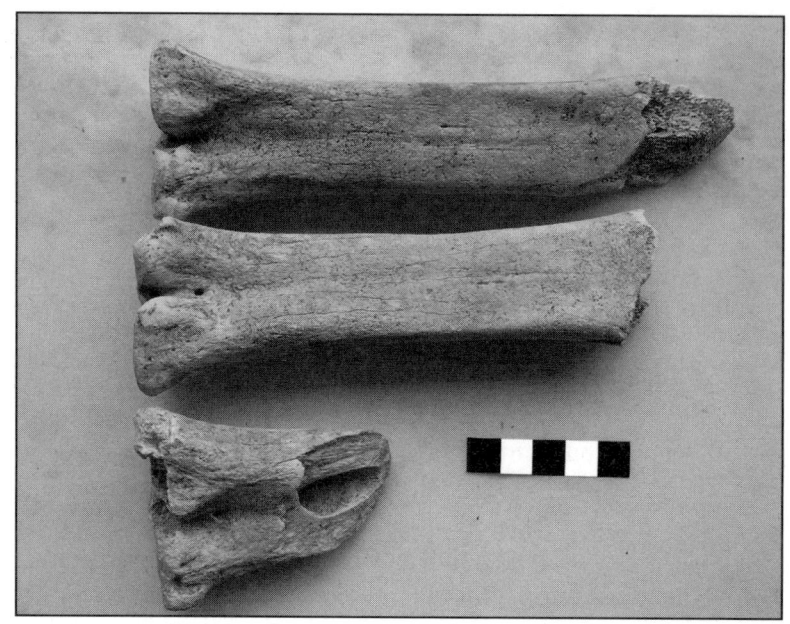

Figure 18.1. Cattle metapodia with distal ends broken off. Photograph K. Harris.

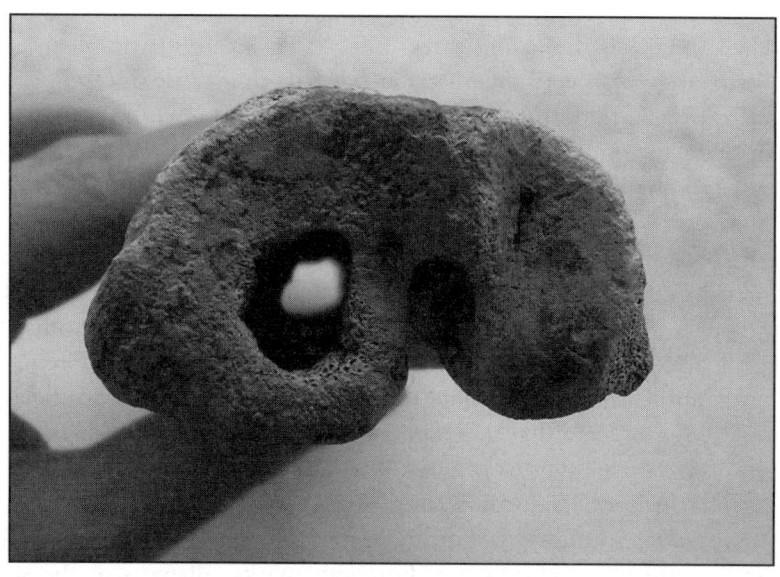

Figure 18.2. Cattle metacarpal with hole in proximal end. Photograph K. Harris.

A Social Zooarchaeology of Feasting: The Evidence from the Ritual Deposit at Nopigeia, Crete

Kerry Harris and Yannis Hamilakis,
University of Southampton

Introduction
This short note summarizes on-going research on an animal bone deposit from Bronze Age Crete which offers the opportunity to comment on the social zooarchaeology of feasting. The deposit comes from a deliberately-dug ditch measuring at least 20m in length and up to 1.5m in depth, dated to the beginning of the Late Bronze Age (*ca.* 1500 BC), a phase known as 'neo-palatial'. Although the ditch is situated close to a long-lived settlement, no architecture has been found associated with it (Vlazaki 1994/6). The material excavated from the ditch consists mostly of several thousands of plain undecorated drinking cups, some cooking vessels and some other forms such as pouring vessels. Many of the cups were found complete, although most were smashed and scattered in the ditch in inter-mixed clusters of pottery and animal bones interspersed with layers of soil. Preliminary soil micromorphological analysis suggests that the backfilling occurred gradually, rather than as one episode (Richard MacPhail n.d.).

The Assemblage
The zooarchaeological material indicates that we are dealing with a special deposit, with a limited range of species of only sheep, goat, pig, cattle and wild goat (*Capra aegagrus cretensis*, agrimi). Some seashells were also found, but concentrated in localized contexts. In general, domestic debris, dogs, equids, a greater variety of wild species, small mammals and birds would also be expected. The total number of fragments identified to species is 995, the Minimum Number of Individuals (MNI) is 44. A minimum of three agrimia were represented, including the deliberate deposition of an impressive agrimi skull with horns on the base of the ditch (at *ca.* 1.5m depth), a basal deposit with meaningful connotations. Of interest is whether this animal was eaten or its presence here is due to its highly symbolic role in Bronze Age Crete, as is often attested iconographically. Animals were deliberately selected from specific age groups: the tooth wear data indicate that sheep/goat were mainly killed at four to six years and pigs between just over one year to just over two years. The evidence for cattle is limited but indicates mature animals; juvenile animals of all species are rare.

Evidence for consumption is indicated by the main meat-bearing bones being well represented and the occurrence of butchery marks; all parts of the skeleton are represented, however, suggesting whole carcasses. There is variation between species: for pig and sheep/goat, the main meat-bearing elements are most commonly represented, whereas for cattle the foot elements were also being utilized. Chop marks are more frequently represented than cut marks and the majority are encountered on the main meat-bearing elements; however chop marks also frequently occur on cattle foot bones. The evidence for burning is minimal but again occurs most frequently on cattle foot bones. This burning is not the result of charring due to roasting meat in open fire; rather it consists of small patches of burning, causing slight discolouration and flaking to the bone surface. This activity facilitates the breaking of these dense bones in order to gain access to the marrow; this can be seen in several cases where the distal end had been broken off (Fig. 18.1) and a hole drilled into the proximal end in order to push the marrow out (Fig. 18.2). Boiling rather than roasting was the main cooking method for meat, a hypothesis supported by the plentiful remnants of tripod cooking pots. The minimal evidence for dog-gnawing and weathering and the presence of articulating elements suggests rapid disposal after consumption.

Conclusion

The importance of this assemblage for analysing zooarchaeologically a feasting assemblage lies in the contextually-bounded nature of the deposit and the association with other feasting paraphernalia such as cooking, eating and drinking vessels. The animal bones represent a selective range of species and ages which were consumed and then ritually deposited and buried. However, its zooarchaeological signature is only partly typical, since meat was most likely boiled rather than roasted, and marrow was extracted from bones and skull, practices not traditionally associated with the ostentatious acts of feasting. This does not necessarily represent a different mode of consumption from the one employed in a domestic, everyday setting. As with the cooking vessels and the thousands of standardized conical cups, it is perhaps not the creation of distinction that is the desired result of this feast but rather one of homogeneity and unity. Importantly, these rituals were characterized by repetition and citation of the past (people were returning to the same spot to perform eating and drinking) and by the deliberate act of burying the remnants. A mnemonic material record of the embodied and sensuous rituals of eating and drinking was thus created, constructing a mnemonic and temporal depth.

Acknowledgements

We would like to thank Dr Maria Vlazaki and the Ephoreia of Prehistoric and Classical Antiquities of West Crete for inviting us to study the material and for facilitating our research; Richard MacPhail for the soil micromorphological research; and the British Academy and the University of Southampton for funding.

References

MacPhail, R. n.d. 'Minoan Crete – ditch fill; assessment of soil micromorphology'. Unpublished report.
Vlazaki, M. 1994/6. 'A prehistoric settlement at Nopigeia, Kisamou', *Kritiki Estia* 5, 11–45 (in Greek).

Fourth-Century AD Glass Tablewares from the Small Bathhouse in Eleutherna-Sector I, Crete

Kalliopi Nikita,
University of Nottingham

Introduction
Glass-blowing revolutionized the manufacture of glass vessels and rapidly commercialized their production in the early first century AD. Owing to their impermeability and transparency glass vessels were transformed into utilitarian commodities, which were available to all social classes throughout the Empire (Harden 1987; Stern 1999, 2001). Despite the ample survival of glass from Roman Crete, its study has been limited (Buechner 1960; Price 1992; Wardle and Wardle 2004), especially as regards material dating after the third century AD (Sternini 1997). The Roman phase (late second to late fourth centuries AD) of the Small Bathhouse in the north-west of Eleutherna-Sector I in north central Crete has yielded a great abundance and diversity of glass vessels, which are the focus of this paper.

Ordinary and Fine Glass Table-wares
A wide range of ordinary and fine table-wares has been identified and dated to the fourth century AD on the basis of typological criteria (Isings 1957; Price 1992; Weinberg 1992) and contextual information (Themelis 2004, 67–69). Free-blowing predominates whereas mould-blowing, engraving, cutting and wheel-abrading occur sporadically. Ordinary wares include various types of cups, beakers, dishes, bowls, jugs, jars, bottles and stemmed goblets of transparent natural bluish and greenish glass. The assemblage also includes an outstanding fine ware consisting of small cups, bowls, saucers, jars and bottles. Their thin-walled, undecorated body was manufactured in colourless free-blown glass. Coils, mostly of translucent turquoise, dark blue, emerald green, and occasionally of amber-brown and purple glass, were applied as ring bases and less often as handles or rims. It seems that this fine bichrome ware is a variation of the trailed-ornament decorative style, which is typical of glass production during the third and fourth centuries AD (Stern 2001, 134; Whitehouse 2001, 138–139).

Archaeological and Technological Considerations
The large assemblages of glass table-wares in the Small Bathhouse of Eleutherna-Sector I, recovered principally from Rooms 58–58b (storerooms) and 65 (shop), reveal that they were intended for serving, consuming, storing and transporting food and drink. Cordials, refreshments or wine, even light repasts were probably offered to the bathers,

as the big volume of cooking-pots, table-wares and utensils in clay and metal also suggest (Themelis 2004, 67–69). It seems that the fine table-wares were to be used by local élites and/or possibly on specific formal occasions. The combined archaeological and technological study of both ordinary and fine table-wares will elucidate various aspects of their technology, manufacture and function in the Bathhouse. Whether these wares were products of a Cretan glass workshop or were associated with an Eastern or a Western production centre is a major question also addressed by using scientific analysis.

References

Buechner, T. S. 1960. 'The glass from Tarrha', *Hesperia* **29** (1), 109–117.

Harden, D. B. 1987. *Glass of the Caesars* (Milan).

Isings, C. 1957. *Roman Glass from Dated Finds* (Groningen).

Price, J. 1992. 'Glass vessels and other objects', in Sackett, L. H. (ed.) *Knossos from the Greek City to Roman Colony, Excavations at the Unexplored Mansion* (London), 415–462.

Stern, E. M. 1999. 'Roman glassblowing in a cultural context', *American Journal of Archaeology* **103**, 441–484.

Stern, E. M. 2001. *Roman, Byzantine and Early Medieval Glass, 10 BCE – 700 CE. Ernesto Wolf Collection* (Ostfildern).

Sternini, M. 1997. 'Vetri', in Di Vita, A. and Martin, A. (eds) *Gortina II. Pretorio il materiale degli scavi Colini 1970–1977* (Padova), 231–263.

Themelis, P. 2004. 'The Polis. East excavation sector I', in Stampolidis, N. C. (ed.) *Eleutherna: Polis, Acropolis, Necropolis* (Athens), 46–80.

Wardle, K. A. and Wardle, D. 2004. 'Glimpses of private life: Roman rock-cut tombs of the first and second centuries AD at Knossos', in Cadogan, G., Hatzaki, E. and Vasilakis, A. (eds) *Knossos: Palace, City, State* (London), 473–480.

Weinberg, G. D. 1992. *Glass Vessels in Ancient Greece: Their History Illustrated from the Collection of the National Museum, Athens* (Athens).

Whitehouse, D. 2001. *Roman Glass in the Corning Museum of Glass, Vol. 2* (New York).

Trout Processing in the Upper Palaeolithic?

Hannah Russ, Randolph Donahue and Andrew Jones, University of Bradford

Introduction
Fish bones have been recovered from six Upper Palaeolithic sites in the Fucino Basin, central Italy (Fig. 20.1). Previous analyses of assemblages from five sites suggested the occurrence of specialized fishing (Wilkens 1994). Recent excavations at Grotta di Pozzo, located in the Fucino Basin area, have recovered a large assemblage of fish bones associated with stone tools and skeletal remains of red deer (*Cervus elaphus*), wild boar (*Sus scrofa*), chamois (*Rupricapra* sp.) and marmot (*Marmota* sp.), all with cut marks (Mussi *et al.* 2004). Fish vertebrae have been dated to 14,650–14,000 cal BP (GX-27906–12,320±50 BP). During this period the Fucino Basin contained a large lake; however, no artefacts linked with fishing have been recovered from any Palaeolithic site in the area. In total 5793 fish bones were retrieved from Grotta di Pozzo. The identifiable remains were all brown trout (*Salmo trutta*). The minimum number (MNI) of trout represented at the site was 133 based on glosso hyal presence. In comparison, only 28 fish were represented by vertebrae.

The high representation of cranial elements compared to vertebrae may suggest that this was a location used for processing fish; however, to assume that these remains result from human exploitation could be very misleading. There are many poorly understood taphonomic processes that potentially affect fish bone assemblages. Fish bones recovered from locations like Grotta di Pozzo, for example, could have been transported by animals such as canids, raptors and ursids. One must distinguish natural and cultural accumulating and modifying agents of fish remains from Palaeolithic sites before they can provide important dietary information of hunter-gatherers and increase understanding of palaeoenvironments.

Previous Research
Important studies by Stewart (1989) and Butler (1990) have developed criteria for distinguishing naturally-accumulated remains from those deposited by humans; however, these criteria are somewhat subjective. Another important aspect is the study of the effects of digestion on fish bones that have passed through the gut of omnivorous species that eat fish (Jones 1984; Nicholson 1993). Macroscopic features of material can be recognized at assemblage level to distinguish between digested and non-digested remains but this is not possible for individual bones. Further research by Evans and Russ (in prep.) indicates that processing fish using stone tools can leave diagnostic traces on fish vertebrae.

Trout Processing in the Upper Palaeolithic?

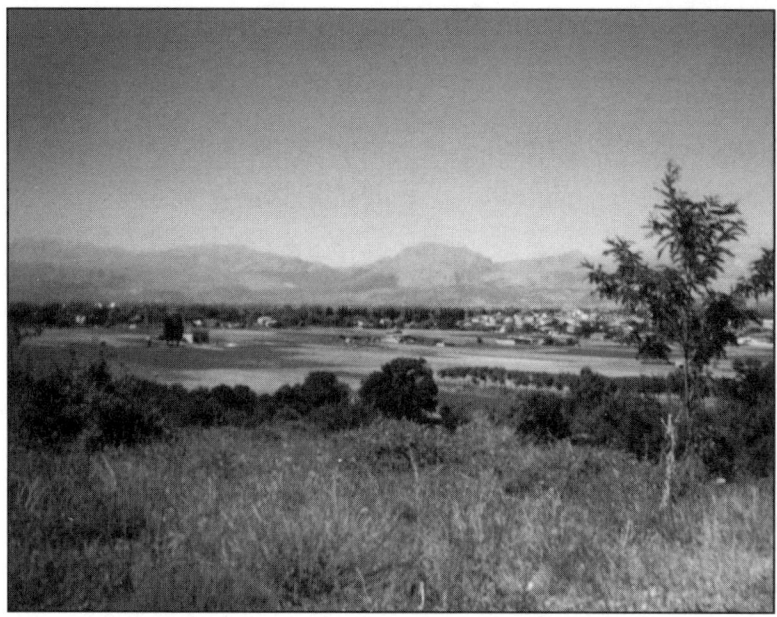

Figure 20.1. The Fucino Basin today. Once the location of Fucine Lake, the basin is now drained for farming. Photograph H. Russ.

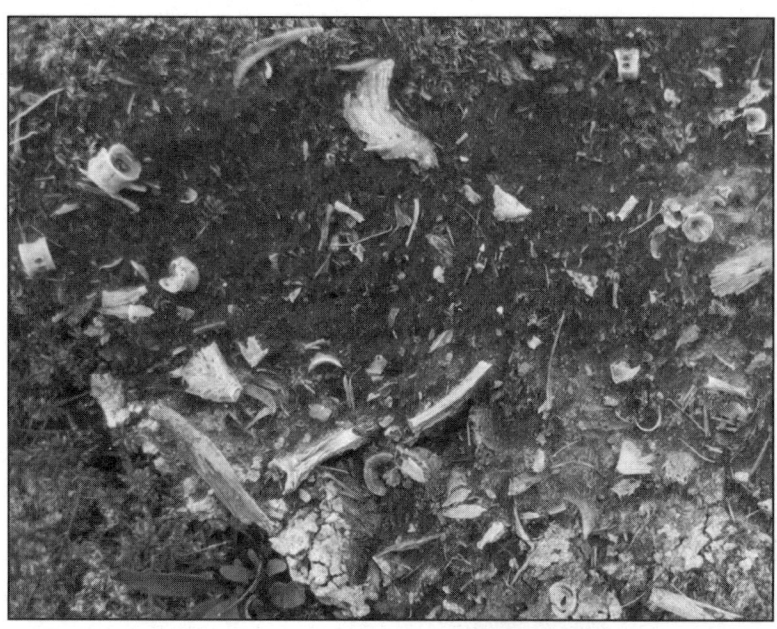

Figure 20.2. Fish remains in a one-year-old bear scat. Photograph R. Smith, Portland State University, USA.

Future Research

To address problems in recognizing human from animal accumulations, further taphonomic and experimental studies are required. An interdisciplinary approach that integrates artefactual and faunal studies, stable isotope analysis, and ethnography with fish bone data will increase resolution for understanding fish exploitation and their material effects by humans and animals in the past. Bones from European archaeological and palaeontological sites ranging from 600,000–10,000 BP will be analysed microscopically to identify surface features that may indicate their agent(s) of accumulation. In addition, experimental material resulting from various processing and cooking techniques based on archaeological and ethnographic evidence will provide microscopic data for recognizing culturally produced assemblages. Faecal and pellet material from non-human mammals (Fig. 20.2) will be dissected to establish the effects of the digestive system for species that are suitable analogues for those of the Palaeolithic.

Acknowledgements

We gratefully acknowledge Professor M. Mussi, University of Rome 'La Sapienza' and Adrian A. Evans, University of Bradford. We would also like to thank Hallo Bay Bear Lodge, Alaska. Financial support from Andy Jagger, Hannah Pickard Funds and the Lithic Microwear Research Laboratory, University of Bradford.

References

Butler, V. L. 1990. *Distinguishing Natural from Cultural Salmonid Deposits in Pacific Northwest North America*, PhD thesis, University of Washington, Seattle.

Evans, A. and Russ, H. in prep. Wear traces on bone and stone.

Jones, A. K. G. 1984. 'Some effects of the mammalian digestive system on fish bones', in Desse-Berset, N. (ed.) *Second Fish Osteoarchaeology Meeting* (Paris), 61–65.

Mussi, M., D'Angelo, E. and Fiore, I. 2004. 'Escargots et autres « petites » ressources alimentaires: le cas de la Grotta di Pozzo (Abruzzes, Italie centrale)', in Brugal, J-P and Desse, J. (eds) *XXIV Rencontres Internationales d'Archéologie et d'Histoire d'Antibes* (Antibes), 99–109.

Nicholson, R. A. 1993. 'An investigation into the effects on fish bone on passage through the human gut: some experiments and comparisons with archaeological material', *Circaea* **10**, 38–51.

Stewart, K. M. 1989. *Fishing Sites of North and East Africa in the Late Pleistocene and Holocene Environmental Change and Human Adaptation* (Oxford).

Wilkens, B. 1994. 'The importance of fishing in the economy of the Fucino Basin (Italy) from Upper Palaeolithic to Neolithic times', *Archaeofauna* **3**, 109–113.

'A People who Eat Wood and Drink Water, the Devil cannot Persuade, nor can Man'. Food in Rural Areas during the Middle Ages (*ca.* AD 1050–1532) in County Dalarna, Sweden: An Example from Västannorstjärn

Mikael Simonsson,
Headland Archaeology Ltd.

Introduction

Situated on the southern border of the topographical and botanical zone called *Limes Norrlandicus* or Lower Norrland in Sweden, lies County Dalarna. The county contains mountain chains in the north and open agricultural landscapes in the south. It is rich in valuable minerals and contains the historically-important mines of East and West Silvberg and Kopparberget at Falun. Dalarna is also one of the most conservative counties in Sweden and new technologies relating to farming were adopted quite late (Selinge 1994, 60; Carlsson 1990, 73; Olsson 1990, 15–17; Berg and Svensson 1969, 7, 9). Today, Dalarna has become the symbol of 'genuine Sweden'. The title for this paper comes from a supposed saying of a Danish bishop describing the people of Dalarna during the fifteenth century.

Dalarna's Middle Ages is generally set between AD 1050 and AD 1523. Dalarna is first mentioned in 1260 as 'The Land of Iron' in Norse sagas and the people are described as pagans. This, combined with archaeological evidence, suggests that the conversion from paganism to Christianity was very slow and was probably not complete until the late thirteenth century (Olsson 1990, 14; Rosén 1993b, 74–81; Nordiska kungasagor 2, 1993, 294; Carlsson 1990, 72). The fact that the medieval kings of Sweden never gained full power over Dalarna has led to the suggestion that a semi-independent community ruled the area (Ersgård 1997, 88). Dalarna was also the focal point for several of Sweden's large-scale peasant rebellions during the fourteenth to sixteenth centuries (Klemming 1866, 25–30; Rosén 1993a, 76).

The Lake of Västannorstjärn

The small village of Västannor is situated in the agriculturally rich area of Häradsbygden. Close to the modern village of Västannor lies the small lake Västannorstjärn which was partly excavated between 1975 and 1978. The excavations revealed a dumping-place for domestic debris, dated by dendrochronology to between AD 1050 and AD 1365 (Landström 1975; Landström 1984, 4, 7). The material consists of over 1000 wooden artefacts, animal bone, leather waste, iron objects and artefacts of silver and glass

'A People who Eat Wood and Drink Water'

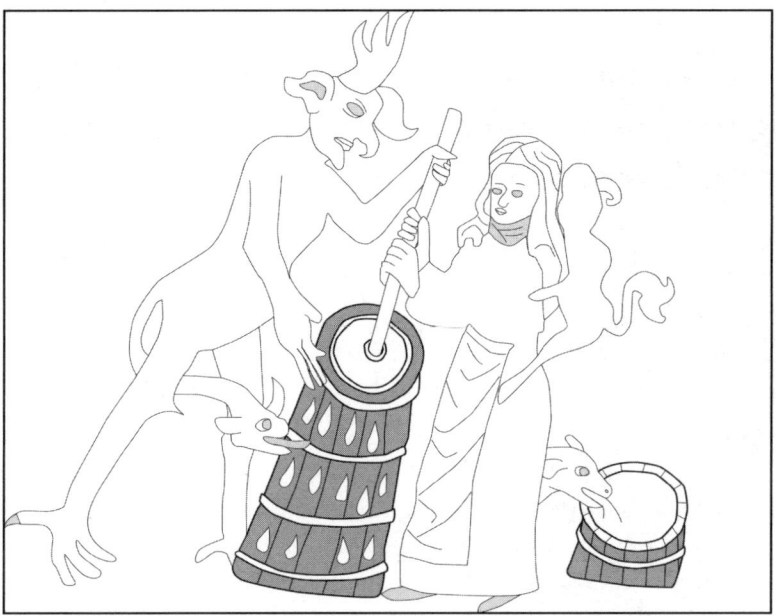

Figure 21.1. There are very few contemporary illustrations showing the processing of dairy products and its artefacts from Sweden. This fifteenth-century depiction from Söderby-Karls church outside Stockholm shows a woman making butter with the help of the Devil, using high and low stave-built vessels. Several staves belonging to vessels like these were discovered during the excavations at Västannorstjärn. Illustration by the author.

(Landström 1984, 7–10; Myrdal 1984, 11–12). The wooden artefacts consist mostly of staves belonging to stave-built vessels, of which over 40 per cent were made of Scots pine. Other wooden objects include rakes, spades, and arrows, fishing equipment, bowls, spoons and oak barrels (Myrdal 1984, 30–31). Studies of the wooden artefacts showed that most of the staves belong to buckets of the same type that have been used until recently in *Limes Norrlandicus* for dairy products, mainly for the creation of '*Långmjölk*', or soured milk (Fig. 21.1). This type of milk is still a very important part of the food culture in Dalarna.

The archaeobotanical samples and pollen cores taken from the lake bed indicate high levels of cereals and an increase in cereal production from the Viking Age onwards (Wennberg and Engelmark 1983 n.d.). Barley is the best represented taxon, with oats and rye being represented occasionally. Few wild berries and herbs were represented, suggesting that the gathering of wild plants was of minor importance.

Analysis of the bone assemblage, which weighed 3.5kg in total, showed sheep/goat to be the dominant taxon, followed by pigs, then cattle (Fig. 21.2). A few fragments of red fox, hare, red squirrel and unidentifiable bird, as well as a possible elk specimen and

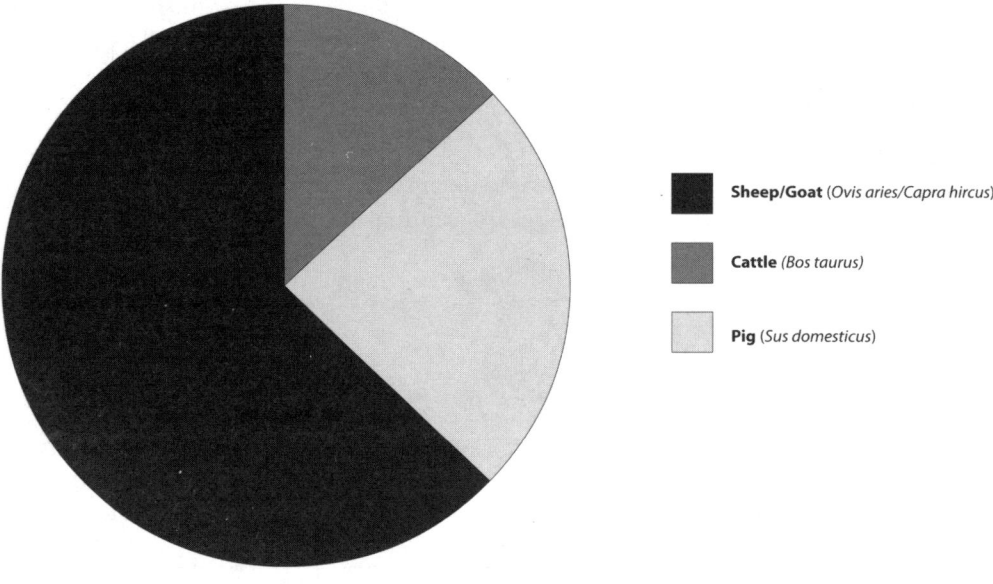

Figure 21.2. Diagram showing the relationship between cattle, sheep/goat and pig at Västannorstjärn. Illustration by the author.

112 bones of fish (mostly pike) were also represented (Arnesson 1979 & 1980). The low frequency of wild mammals suggests that game made little contribution to the diet, although it is clear from finds of arrows that hunting did take place. The representation of red fox and red squirrel suggest that wild animals were exploited mainly for fur, something that corresponds very well with animal bone assemblages from other medieval dwellings in Dalarna. The relative abundance of fish bones, combined with the discovery of fishing-related artefacts (hooks and net sinks), suggests that fish were an important part of the diet. That most of the bones were from pike indicates that fishing concentrated on the lake itself. However, the discovery of oak barrel staves (oak does not grow in the region) suggests that fish, probably salted herring, were also imported to the village.

Conclusion

From the available data it is possible to reconstruct diet at Västannorstjärn and in *Limes Norrlandicus* during the Middle Ages, and ultimately to enhance our understanding of everyday life in this area.

It is clear that the diet in Västannorstjärn was based on barley, possibly in the form of porridge, beer and bread, together with dairy products, most likely in the form of '*Långmjölk*'. Meat was consumed, but only that from sheep, goat and pig was eaten regularly. Fish, both locally-caught and imported, may actually have been more important than meat. Other wild animals were also exploited but probably more for their fur than their meat, although the bones from wild birds suggest that these were eaten occasionally.

The picture of consumption practices at Västannorstjärn is very different from the stereotypical diet assumed for Sweden in the Middle Ages: the inhabitants of the Land of Iron seem to have consumed fish, porridge and dairy products, rather than the traditional 'meat and beer' diet of medieval Scandinavia.

Acknowledgements

I wish to thank Greger Bennström, Ewa Carlsson Fredrik Sandberg and Anna Lögdqvist at the County Museum of Dalarna Archaeological Unit, Dr Jonas Monie Nordin at the University of Stockholm for all the help in relation to my Master thesis at the University of Lund in 2005. I also would like to direct my gratitude and thanks to Dr Anders Ödman, Lecturer in Medieval Archaeology at the University of Lund, for all the encouragement and help I received during the research.

References

Arnesson, A. 1979. *Osteologisk Undersökning av Benmaterialet från Boplatsen Västannortjärn, Leksands sn, Dalarna.* Unpublished script, Stockholm University.

Arnesson, A. 1980. *Totalt Västannortjärn, Leksands sn, Dalarna.* Unpublished script

Berg, G. and Svensson, S. 1969. *Svensk Bondekultur* (Stockholm).

Carlsson, E. 1990. *Medeltiden. Ca 1050–1520. Alla tiders landskap. Riksintresse för kulturmiljövården i Kopparbergs län. Dalarnas hembygdsbok 1990* (Falun).

Ersgård, L. 1997. *Det Starka Landskapet: En Arkeologisk Studie av Leksandsbygden i Dalarna från yngre järnålder till nyare tid* (Stockholm).

Klemming, G- E. 1866. *Svenska Medeltidens Rimkrönikor. Efter en Originalhandskrift Utgifven av G. E. Klemming. D. 2, Nya eller Karls-krönikan: Början av unionsstriderna samt Karl Knutssons regering, 1389–1452* (Stockholm).

Landström, K.-H. 1975. *Västannortjärn, Leksands Socken, Dalarna. Rapport över 1975 års undersökningar.* Dalarna Museum Dn 258/75.

Landström, K.-H. 1984. *Den Arkeologiska Undersökningen. Vardagsliv i en Medeltida Bondby. Fynd från Västannortjärn i Leksand, Dalarna* (Leksand).

Myrdal, J 1984. *Träföremålen. Vardagsliv i en medeltida bondby. Fynd från Västannortjärn i Leksand, Dalarna. Red. Myrdal, J. Leksands kommun* (Leksand).

Nordiska kungasagor 2. *Olav den Heliges Saga* (Trondheim).

Olsson, D. S. 1990. *Bebyggelselandskapet i Dalarna: Alla Tiders Landskap. Riksintresse för kulturmiljövården i Kopparbergs län. Dalarnas hembygdsbok 1990* (Falun).

Rosén, J. 1993a. *Engelbrekt och unionen, uppror och förhandlingar 1434–1441. Den Svenska historien, tredje bandet. Kyrka och riddarliv. Karl Knutsson och Sturetiden* (Stockholm).

Rosén, J. 1993b. *Oppositionen mot Gustav Vasa 1523–1531. Den Svenska historien, fjärde bandet. Gustav Vasa. Riket formas* (Stockholm).

Selinge, K.-G. 1994. *National Atlas of Sweden: Cultural Heritage and Preservation* (Stockholm).

Wennberg, B. and Engelmark, R. 1983. *Preliminär Rapport över frön och frukter från Västannortjärn, Leksand sn, Dalarna.* Unpublished script.